MW00910704

Public Health Tools for Practicing Psychologists

About the Authors

Jalie A. Tucker, PhD, MPH, is Professor and Chair of the Department of Health Behavior in the School of Public Health at the University of Alabama at Birmingham (UAB) and directs the UAB Addictive Behaviors and Health Studies group. She earned a doctorate in clinical psychology in 1979 (Vanderbilt University) and an MPH in health care organization and policy in 1998 (UAB). Dr. Tucker's research interests include the behavioral economics of substance misuse, help-seeking, and behavior change, including how positive change occurs with and without clinical treatment. Dr. Tucker has authored or coauthored numerous journal articles and book chapters and has been a coeditor of two books, including *Changing Additive Behavior: Bridging Clinical and Public Health Strategies* (1999). She is a past president of the Division on Addictions (50) of the American Psychological Association (APA), a past member and chair of the APA Board of Professional Affairs, and a four-term APA Council of Representatives member.

Diane M. Grimley, PhD, is Professor in the Department of Health Behavior in the School of Public Health at the University of Alabama at Birmingham. She earned a doctorate in health psychology in 1994 (University of Rhode Island). Dr. Grimley's research interests include STD/HIV and other reproductive health issues, multiple health risk behaviors, and theory-based, technology-delivered behavioral interventions. Dr. Grimley has authored or coauthored numerous journal articles and has served on the editorial board of *AIDS and Behavior*. She is currently on the editorial board of *Sexually Transmitted Diseases* and the *American Journal of Health Behavior*. She also serves on the Advisory Board of *Public Health Reports*, published by the American Schools of Public Health (ASPH).

Advances in Psychotherapy – Evidence-Based Practice

Series Editor
Danny Wedding, PhD, MPH, Professor of Psychology, California School of Professional Psychology / Alliant International University, San Francisco, CA

Associate Editors
Larry Beutler, PhD, Professor, Palo Alto University / Pacific Graduate School of Psychology, Palo Alto, CA
Kenneth E. Freedland, PhD, Professor of Psychiatry and Clinical Health Psychology, Washington University School of Medicine, St. Louis, MO
Linda C. Sobell, PhD, ABPP, Professor, Center for Psychological Studies, Nova Southeastern University, Ft. Lauderdale, FL
David A. Wolfe, PhD, RBC Chair in Children's Mental Health, Centre for Addiction and Mental Health, University of Toronto, ON

The basic objective of this series is to provide therapists with practical, evidence-based treatment guidance for the most common disorders seen in clinical practice – and to do so in a "reader-friendly" manner. Each book in the series is both a compact "how-to-do" reference on a particular disorder for use by professional clinicians in their daily work, as well as an ideal educational resource for students and for practice-oriented continuing education.
The most important feature of the books is that they are practical and "reader-friendly:" All are structured similarly and all provide a compact and easy-to-follow guide to all aspects that are relevant in real-life practice. Tables, boxed clinical "pearls", marginal notes, and summary boxes assist orientation, while checklists provide tools for use in daily practice.

Public Health Tools for Practicing Psychologists

Jalie A. Tucker and Diane M. Grimley
School of Public Health, University of Alabama at Birmingham, AL

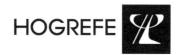

Library of Congress Cataloging in Publication

is available via the Library of Congress Marc Database under the
Library of Congress Control Number 2010935193

Library and Archives Canada Cataloguing in Publication

Tucker, Jalie A. (Jalie Ann), 1954-
    Public health tools for practicing psychologists / Jalie A. Tucker and Diane M. Grimley.

(Advances in psychotherapy--evidence-based practice ; v. 20) Includes bibliographical references.
ISBN 978-0-88937-330-3

    1. Mental health services. I. Grimley, Diane M.
II. Title. III. Series: Advances in
psychotherapy--evidence-based practice ; v. 20

RA790.T83 2010   362.1   C2010-905708-2

© 2011 by Hogrefe Publishing

PUBLISHING OFFICES
USA: Hogrefe Publishing, 875 Massachusetts Avenue, 7th Floor, Cambridge, MA 02139
                Phone (866) 823-4726, Fax (617) 354-6875; E-mail customerservice@hogrefe-publishing.com
EUROPE: Hogrefe Publishing, Rohnsweg 25, 37085 Göttingen, Germany
                Phone +49 551 49609-0, Fax +49 551 49609-88, E-mail publishing@hogrefe.com

SALES & DISTRIBUTION
USA: Hogrefe Publishing, Customer Services Department,
                30 Amberwood Parkway, Ashland, OH 44805
                Phone (800) 228-3749, Fax (419) 281-6883, E-mail customerservice@hogrefe.com
EUROPE: Hogrefe Publishing, Rohnsweg 25, 37085 Göttingen, Germany
                Phone +49 551 49609-0, Fax +49 551 49609-88, E-mail publishing@hogrefe.com

OTHER OFFICES
CANADA: Hogrefe Publishing, 660 Eglinton Ave. East, Suite 119-514, Toronto, Ontario, M4G 2K2
SWITZERLAND: Hogrefe Publishing, Länggass-Strasse 76, CH-3000 Bern 9

Hogrefe Publishing
Incorporated and registered in the Commonwealth of Massachusetts, USA, and in Göttingen, Lower Saxony,
Germany

No part of this book may be reproduced, stored in a retrieval system or transmitted, in any form or by any means,
electronic, mechanical, photocopying, microfilming, recording or otherwise, without written permission from the
publisher.

Printed and bound in the USA
ISBN: 978-0-88937-330-3

Preface

In 2009, the US National Institutes of Health (NIH) convened an institute-wide meeting on the science of behavior change (SOBC) to aid development of a roadmap for behavior change research (see http://nihroadmap.nih.gov/documents/SOBC_Meeting_Summary_2009.pdf). Attendees were a multidisciplinary group of invited experts and NIH staff from 17 institutes. Major themes included: (1) Individual- and population-level approaches should be better linked in multilevel strategies to promote healthy behaviors in order to have broader public health impact; (2) Understanding factors that shape health decision-making and the environmental contexts of choice are vital to developing effective change strategies, and span applications of ecological models, behavioral economics, and social network analysis, among others; (3) Health risk behaviors cluster in bundles that need to be targeted simultaneously; and (4) New methods and measures are needed that support assessment of multilevel, contextually framed trajectories of behavior change and that can serve as cost-effective platforms for population-scale interventions (e.g., mobile phones). The overall conclusion was that "The science of behavior change has long suffered from fragmentation along scientific and topical boundaries. . . . Because unhealthy behaviors cause so much morbidity and mortality, the status quo cannot prevail" (NIH, 2009, pp. 5–6).

The same forces operating to produce this visionary NIH roadmap for SOBC research are at play in the content of this book, which is concerned with providing psychologists with new tools from public health to motivate and maintain behavior change. The methods discussed are rooted in the same evidence base that sparked the SOBC meeting. They are meant to supplement, not replace, the longstanding emphasis of psychological practice on treating individuals for a focal disorder using the tools of psychotherapy.

The book aims to make a modest contribution to the dissemination process that brings evidence-based innovations to the attention of front-line providers, in this case from the science and practice of public health as it intersects with mental health, substance misuse, and other health behavior problems of interest to psychologists. Psychologists have been at the forefront of developing the SOBC knowledge base. We believe they likewise have much to contribute to a broadened "integrated behavioral health care" practice agenda that maintains a degree of individualization of care, in concert with dissemination strategies from public health. Such an integrated approach to care will reach more persons in need who could benefit from services for psychological and behavioral problems, ultimately enhancing the public's well-being and overall quality of life.

Acknowledgments

We are grateful to Linda Sobell, PhD, ABPP, Series Associate Editor, for creating the opportunity for us to describe the tools of public health practice for our psychology colleagues as part of the Hogrefe/APA Division 12 series *Advances in Psychotherapy – Evidence-Based Practice*. Serendipity played a role in that the idea for the book was formulated when Linda Sobell and J.A.T. were seated together at the American Psychological Association Council of Representatives meeting in February 2007. Linda and J.A.T., along with coauthor D.M.G., share a longstanding interest in broadening the scope of psychological practice in the direction of public health that builds on the profession's clinical bedrock. Series Editor Danny Wedding, PhD, MPH, also shares a background in public health and supported the book's development and placement as part of the series, even though it deviates from the usual focus on evidence-based treatments for specific disorders. We thank Robert Dimbleby of Hogrefe Publishing for his support of the project. We also thank our colleagues at the UAB School of Public Health, Cathy A. Simpson, PhD, and Susan D. Chandler, MPH, who cheerfully provided expert content input and editing as we drafted the book. Dr. Simpson provided the case vignette for Chapter 5 that illustrates how the tools of clinical and public health practice can be assembled in an integrated system of behavioral health care, in this case for persons living with HIV/AIDS in a rural, disadvantaged region of Alabama. Finally, we are indebted to the pioneering masters in our field who touched our professional lives at a "teachable moment" and inspired us to see the possibilities of expanding our clinical world view in the direction of public health. J.A.T. thanks G. Alan Marlatt and David B. Abrams, and D.M.G. thanks James O. Prochaska.

Dedication

To my mother Helen Hutchison Tucker, who gave me the gift of curiosity.
JAT

To my loving children, James W. Grimley and Heather M. Miller.
DMG

Introduction:
The Changing Practice Environment

Psychologists and other mental health practitioners have historically focused on the individual as the primary consumer of services, typically in the form of psychological assessment and psychotherapy. Although individual clinical practice remains an important professional activity, the scope, target, and types of mental health services continue to evolve and expand as the broader health care environment in which psychological services are delivered changes. In addition to an enduring focus on mental health treatment for persons who seek clinical care, there is increasing concern with providing services to the larger population of persons with problems that do not seek care. This untreated population segment contributes the bulk of harm and cost related to mental health and substance use (MH/SU) problems, and a large gap exists between the need for and utilization of services (US Surgeon General, 1999; Wang, Lane, Olfson, Pincus, Wells, & Kessler, 2005). In addition to clinical treatment, essential services include preventive or limited therapeutic services for persons with less serious problems and programs that facilitate behavior patterns to promote health and prevent illness. This expanded *"behavioral health"* agenda encompasses physical and mental health and targets individuals, communities, and health systems, including improving access to quality, evidence-based care.

> **"Behavioral health" services encompass physical and mental health and target broader constituencies than individual psychotherapy.**

Mental health practitioners have much to contribute to this agenda, but doing so requires adopting a broader perspective on psychological services and learning new tools for practice that come from other fields, including public health. This book provides basic knowledge about public health perspectives on mental health and introduces practitioners to public health practices and advances in communications technology that can be used to extend the reach and impact of psychological services.

Several forces have converged to promote an expansion of services. These include the rapidly changing health care environment, the associated evidence-based practice (EBP) movement, and efforts to de-stigmatize MH/SU disorders and to make treatment more accessible (Institute of Medicine [IOM], 2006; US Surgeon General, 1999). In the late 20th century, health care became an industry obsessed with containing costs, and independent fee-for-service practice involving a single provider and patient gave way to more complex service delivery arrangements epitomized by managed care organizations (MCOs) (Mechanic, 1994). Mental health services were increasingly delivered either by nonspecialist providers in primary medical care or by specialist providers in "behavioral health carve-outs" that typically required prior approval by MCO gatekeepers (Cummings, O'Donohue, & Ferguson, 2003; IOM, 2006).

Federal parity legislation in 1996 and 2008 expanded coverage of services for MH/SU disorders in ways that began to approximate coverage of comparable medical care. These changes helped expand coverage of MH/SU services and moved some services into mainstream medical practice, thereby reducing stigma (e.g., for depression and its treatment). For example, the US Medicaid program now offers reimbursement for alcohol and drug screening and brief interventions. However, specialty care for extended periods has been abridged, often with adverse effects on access and outcomes, particularly for the seriously mentally ill (Mechanic, 1994). Moreover, improved MH/SU benefits enacted by parity legislation are likely to be superseded in the United States by the US Patient Protection and Affordable Care Act of 2010 that reaffirms parity requirements and increases coverage of mental health care through Medicare and Medicaid (American Psychological Association, 2010). This complex legislation has a long lead-in time, however, so the future impact on behavioral health services remains ambiguous at present.

> **Third-party-payer coverage has expanded, but time limits are common.**

Concurrent with these changes, the EBP movement developed as a means of promoting scientifically guided, patient-focused quality care in health systems that are increasingly regulated and organizationally and financially complex (IOM, 2001, 2006). These trends almost certainly will continue as US federal health care reforms are enacted over the next decade.

Collectively, these forces operating on the practice environment have led to a broadened conception of psychological services that encompasses, but is not limited to, individual-based clinical assessment and treatment. The modal client for many psychologists is no longer the self-referred, motivated outpatient psychotherapy client who can be assessed extensively and then treated for as long as the therapist and client consider necessary and desirable for continued improvement. Psychological services are increasingly limited in number and duration by MCOs and other third-party payers, and interventions that involve fewer sessions and less intensive and more focused therapeutic approaches are becoming the norm for many uncomplicated problems. Furthermore, psychologists are working more with medical patients and other persons who do not view themselves as having psychological issues, who are not aware of how their behavior may be affecting their health, and who are not particularly motivated to make changes (Cummings et al., 2003).

> **Behavioral health services span a broad range of needs, including prevention, early intervention, and intensive treatment of serious illness.**

The conventional tools of psychotherapeutic practice are not well suited to delivering the range of services needed in this complex practice environment. Although psychotherapy will remain an essential element of psychologists' repertoire, an expanded skill set and approach to service delivery are needed to meet the demands of the contemporary health care environment. This book is about one such avenue open to psychologists to expand their skills and services: namely, how to bring the tools of public health into psychological practice in ways that complement and expand clinical approaches, thereby reaching more people in need with services that are appropriately varied in scope and intensity.

This has long been a goal of good group health plans, which offer a range of services and seek to match the type and level of care to patient needs. Our contention is that psychologists can serve a larger, more heterogeneous client base by diversifying their services through integration of basic public health and clinical strategies. This integrated approach represents an exciting advance in behavioral health practice and adds new methods to the arsenal of practicing psychologists well-versed in clinical methods.

> **This book describes an integrative approach to expanding clinical practice, based on a public health or population perspective.**

This book is intended to offer psychologists and other mental health professionals new ways to expand their practice by introducing them to basic philosophies, concepts, and intervention approaches in public health. Public health principles and methods, such as market segmentation, identifying "teachable moments," and delivering motivationally congruent messages to risk groups, will be described with illustrative examples that span low- to high-technology applications. The role of screening and brief interventions (SBIs) in behavioral health care will be discussed, followed by low-technology interventions that use print materials, videos, DVDs, and other self-change materials. Then, interventions that use communications and computer technologies are described, including interactive voice response (IVR) systems that are particularly useful for monitoring and supporting behavior change over long intervals for chronic problems that remit and relapse (Abu-Hasaballah, James, & Aseltine, 2007). Other applications involve the use of cell phones and computers to facilitate automated, tailored interventions that maintain an individualized or client-centered approach to behavior change while capturing the broad reach of public health (Kreuter, Farrell, Olevitch, & Brennan, 2000).

Table of Contents

1

Description

1.1 Terminology

This section introduces concepts, terms, and intervention approaches from public health and contrasts them with clinical approaches. Understanding how the approaches differ and complement one another is basic to effective integration.

1.1.1 Clinical and Public Health Practice Models

Until recently, interventions for promoting psychological well-being and behavioral health tended to be either individual or small-group intensive clinical treatments delivered by mental health specialists, or large-scale public health programs delivered to at-risk populations, such as school-based programs (e.g., the President's Challenge Youth Physical Fitness Awards and Project D.A.R.E. [Drug Abuse Resistance Education]). Clinical interventions generally are client-centered, individualized, and delivered to motivated individuals who seek care. They tend to have greater benefits in reducing risk behaviors on a per-person basis than do public health interventions, which typically are generic, less intensive and costly per person, and delivered to a heterogeneous audience. However, clinical interventions reach only the small subset of persons who reactively seek services, whereas public health interventions generally have broad reach into the population in need. This reach is achieved via proactive intervention delivery to large numbers of people who are not otherwise seeking services.

> Clinical interventions generally achieve greater risk reduction for individuals, but population approaches reach more people in need.

1.1.2 Population Impact of Practice Approaches

Recent work integrates public health and clinical strategies in order to target larger risk groups with interventions that are individualized, at least in part, thereby increasing the potential overall *impact* of services on population health. Advances in computer and communication technologies have helped to combine the best of clinical and public health strategies so that large segments of the population in need can be reached with individualized interventions. Concurrently, behavior change theories and techniques have broadened to support proactive recruitment and intervention delivery to less motivated persons who are not reactively seeking services.

These advances in behavior change theories and techniques, in concert with information technology, have increased the scope and potential public health

Combining clinical and population approaches achieves the greatest impact. Impact = Reach × Efficacy.

impact of behavior change programs. Impact is defined as the product of the intervention's reach, or the percentage of individuals who receive the intervention, and its efficacy, or the percentage of individuals who show a defined benefit, that is: impact = reach × efficacy (Abrams & Emmons, 1997). Table 1 illustrates the concept of impact as it applies to clinical, public health, and integrated approaches to behavioral health care that vary in their reach and efficacy. The text box describes intervention "efficacy," an essential determinant of population impact, and its companion concept of intervention "effectiveness."

Public health interventions are typically generic, less intensive and costly than clinical treatments, and can reach more persons in need.

Although distinctions between clinical and public health approaches have blurred somewhat in recent years, clinical interventions tend to be more intensive, costly, efficacious, and "higher threshold" in that they require entry into the health care system. Public health interventions can be disseminated more widely to target audiences in the broader community. They tend to be generic and typically are less intensive, costly, and efficacious on a per-person basis. Clinical interventions require active help-seeking on the part of recipients. In contrast, public health programs actively target recipients who often are not motivated to seek services. As shown in Table 1, a more efficacious individual-level intervention may have lower overall impact than a less efficacious public health intervention that reaches many more people. For example, whereas hospital-based alcohol treatment for one alcohol-dependent patient may cost in excess of US $10,000, for about US $70,000, a health care organization could implement alcohol screening and brief intervention with about 10,000 adults (Fleming et al., 2002). Thus, well-conducted integrated behavioral health programs have potential for greater population impact compared with clinical

Table 1
Impact of Behavioral Interventions With Varying Reach and Efficacy

Intervention approach	Practice target and methods	% Population Reached	Efficacy (% improved)	Population impact
Clinical	One-on-one or small group; 6-12 visits; reactive health care	5	30	1.5
Public health	Community-population based; mass media delivery; proactive	90	2	1.6
Integrated	Community/population; technology-assisted, individualized interventions; proactive, targeted	60	20	12.0

Note. Adapted from "Health Behavior and Health Education: The Past, Present, and Future," by D. B. Abrams, & K. M. Emmons, in Health Behavior and Health Education: Theory, Research, and Practice, K. Glanz., B. K. Rimer, & F. M. Lewis, Eds., 1997, San Francisco, CA: Jossey-Bass, pp. 453–478.

Intervention Efficacy and Effectiveness

The terms *efficacy* and *effectiveness* both relate to the basic question in evaluation research: "Did an intervention work?" However, they address different questions along the continuum of decision-making about the strength, meaning, and generalizability of research findings. Borrowing from Flay's (1986) analysis, *efficacy trials* evaluate whether an intervention does more good than harm when delivered under optimum conditions, as in a well-resourced randomized controlled trial (RCT). In an efficacy trial, participants with pure forms of a disorder who are motivated to comply can be selected for inclusion; treatment and control conditions can be implemented with high fidelity; and outcomes are assessed on a preplanned follow-up schedule. These design features promote high internal validity, but the generalization of findings to more diverse populations in less well controlled and resourced settings may be limited.

Effectiveness trials evaluate whether an intervention does more good than harm under real-world conditions of availability, implementation, and utilization (Flay, 1986). Participants tend to be more heterogeneous along demographic and disorder-relevant dimensions, including having comorbid conditions that may adversely affect outcomes. Intervention and follow-up procedures may be implemented less consistently, and randomization to treatment or control conditions may be impractical or unethical. Effectiveness studies thus may have lower internal validity than efficacy studies, but they tend to have higher external validity. They contribute important information about the extent to which an intervention can be successfully translated into routine practice.

Ideally, an intervention established as efficacious in RCTs will be evaluated in usual practice or community settings to determine whether it provides benefits under less well controlled conditions. Effectiveness studies that do not involve random assignment allow investigation of how extratherapeutic patient and contextual variables may affect outcomes; e.g., how do the environmental circumstances that surround treatment-seeking affect treatment engagement, retention, and outcomes? Such extratherapeutic factors influence behavior change and can be studied better in effectiveness than efficacy trials.

or public health approaches alone. Integrated behavioral health care typically involves some degree of individualization that can improve efficacy on a per-person basis, coupled with dissemination concepts and strategies pioneered in public health practice to reach more persons in need.

Integrated behavioral health care combines some degree of tailoring with public health dissemination strategies to increase reach into the community.

1.1.3   Developing an Intervention Spectrum

An emerging strategy is to combine public health, integrated behavioral health, and clinical care in a coordinated service delivery system that encompasses prevention and treatment and allocates limited helping resources based on population and individual need and risk. Figure 1 shows a population-based allocation scheme adapted from an early IOM (1994) model to broaden MH/SU clinical services in the direction of prevention. As the figure shows, a far greater proportion of the population will need and benefit from preventive interventions compared with the minority in need of treatment-related services that range from initial case-finding, to acute treatment, to long-term care.

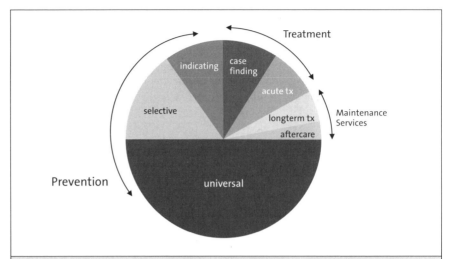

Figure 1
System of care spanning the intervention spectrum for psychological and behavioral disorders. Proportions in the pie graph reflect segments of the population that need and can benefit from different interventions ranging from universal prevention to posttreatment aftercare. Tx = treatment. Adapted from *Reducing Risks for Mental Disorders: Frontiers for Preventive Intervention Research*, by the Institute of Medicine, 1994, Washington, DC: National Academies Press, p. 23.

Within the prevention sector, approaches can include *universal, selective,* or *indicated prevention* (IOM, 1994). This range encompasses interventions that are increasingly intensive and targeted to specific at-risk recipients. Universal prevention programs target the general public or population without regard to individual risk factors (e.g., television campaigns to "Get Five Daily" to increase general population intake of fruits and vegetables). Selective preventive interventions target population subgroups or individuals who have above-average risk factors for a preventable or treatable disorder (e.g., campaigns aimed at older women advocating bone density screenings). Indicated prevention interventions target individuals who have detectable but "subclinical" symptoms and signs for a disorder that typically fall short of clinical diagnosis (e.g., physician guidance on nutrition and weight management based on early signs of metabolic syndrome). Brief screening programs of at-risk population segments support "case-finding" of persons who meet some or all diagnostic criteria and who may benefit from preventive or clinical interventions. Ideally, case-finding will occur early in problem development before a disorder is established and serious and, therefore, more difficult to treat.

> **Prevention can be universal, selective, or indicated.**

Traditionally, most mental health practitioners have limited their services to acute or intensive treatment such as time-limited psychotherapy and the assessment procedures that support it. Although most practitioners will not participate across the full intervention spectrum outlined by the IOM (1994), there are many feasible opportunities and tools to expand their scope of practice. The first is to expand practice activities beyond the clinical treatment sector in the direction of indicated and selective preventive interventions, and case-finding in non-treatment-seeking individuals and at-risk subgroups. The second is to provide "extensive" services over long intervals that are fairly

> **Practice can be expanded by offering low-intensity, long-term "extensive" services in addition to traditional intensive therapies.**

RE-AIM Framework for Behavioral Health Evaluations

The scope of assessment tends to be broader when behavioral health interventions are evaluated compared with the psychotherapy outcome literature familiar to mental health practitioners. The RE-AIM framework is emerging as a way to evaluate the real-world impact of behavioral health interventions (Glasgow, Klesges, Dzewaltowski, Estabrooks, & Vogt, 2006). The framework evaluates an intervention on five factors: **R**each (the proportion of the target population that receives the intervention), **E**fficacy (success rate or positive outcomes), **A**doption (the number of settings, practices, or health plans that use the intervention), **I**mplementation (the number of times the intervention is implemented as intended), and **M**aintenance (the extent or duration to which an intervention is sustained over time). These five factors in combination determine the public health impact or population-based effects of an intervention. Although not yet a publication requirement for research evaluations, the RE-AIM framework is a useful way to plan and evaluate behavioral health interventions.

---

minimal and supportive in scope (Humphreys & Tucker, 2002). Such services offer long-term monitoring of chronic relapsing and remitting disorders (e.g., addictive disorders) with linkages to care when problems reemerge.

This book focuses on these sectors where abundant opportunities exist to expand psychological practice. An optimal continuum of care will offer a range of services and will facilitate consumer-selected and professionally recommended choices in ways that maximize individual and aggregate benefits on behavioral health (Tucker & Simpson, in press). Evaluation of such services will similarly need to be broader than the usual focus on individual outcomes of psychotherapy. The text box describes an approach to evaluation research that is common in public health, the RE-AIM framework, and illustrates key evaluation questions for real-world interventions that seek to change individual behavior and to have an impact on population behavioral health.

> The ideal continuum of care covers a spectrum of services, encourages consumer involvement, and maximizes individual and population health benefits.

1.2   Definitions

Integrated behavioral health care depends on adopting a *population perspective*. A basic orienting assumption is that systems of care should offer a range of services of varying scope and intensity, corresponding to the range of needs and preferences in the population (Humphreys & Tucker, 2002). This means attending to and serving the needs of the larger population segment that does not seek services and tends to have less severe problems, in addition to the minority segment that presents for clinical care and tends to have more serious problems. For many disorders, the larger untreated segment with less serious problems overall contributes the bulk of harm and cost at the population level.

> A population perspective argues for offering a range of services for different levels of need and consumer preferences.

Reducing barriers to care and developing a continuum of appealing, accessible services are public health priorities in this endeavor (Tucker & Simpson, in press). Doing so depends on understanding the needs, preferences, and barriers to care for the underserved majority (e.g., Tucker, Foushee, & Simpson, 2009). These issues can be addressed using the tools of *social marketing*

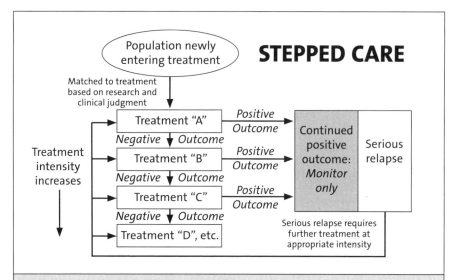

Figure 2
A stepped care approach to the delivery of health care services. Based on "Treatment for problem drinkers: A public health priority," by M. B. Sobell & L. C. Sobell, in J. S. Baer, G. A. Marlatt, & R. J. McMahon, Eds., 1993, *Addictive Behaviors Across the Lifespan: Prevention, Treatment, and Policy Issues,* Beverly Hills, CA: Sage, p. 150.

(Weinreich, 1999). High-risk groups, or "market segments," are offered interventions tailored to address their specific problems and preferences. As discussed later in Chapter 3, effective market segmentation may use consumer surveys or focus groups to assess the needs, preferences, strengths, and resources of potential target groups. Interventions then can be devised accordingly, as discussed in Chapter 4.

A related strategy known as "stepped care" is shown in Figure 2. Stepped care entails using the least intensive and least costly intervention that is effective as the first line of service delivery, rather than initially offering everyone the most intensive (and often most costly) treatment (Sobell & Sobell, 2000). If a less intensive approach is not sufficient, care can be "stepped up" and intensified. Stepped care approaches are common in medicine and help spread limited health care resources to more individuals using a rational needs-based approach. For example, many individuals with uncomplicated behavior problems show significant improvements after brief motivational interventions involving one to two sessions (Miller & Rollnick, 2002). Extended psychotherapy is unnecessary and should be reserved for persons with complex, serious, and comorbid disorders.

Collectively, this approach involves a spectrum of "low- to high-threshold" services of variable intensity and professional involvement. Examples of lower threshold services include guided self-change programs that individuals use on their own; screening and brief interventions (SBIs); *telehealth* options that use phone and computer systems to extend the reach of care; and automated expert systems that tailor individual "behavioral prescriptions" based on detailed assessment information. These services can be delivered opportunistically and

Social marketing addresses the needs, preferences, and barriers to care among potential consumers of services.

Stepped care begins with the least intensive service and ramps up to more intensive treatments if initial services prove inadequate.

Lower threshold services include guided self-change, screening and brief intervention, telehealth, and behavioral "prescriptions."

proactively through outreach efforts to risk groups or individuals with risk factors in community or nonspecialty medical settings, instead of waiting for them to reactively seek services. If such services are readily available (e.g., outside the health care system or via "treatment on demand" arrangements), people can access them quickly when their motivation shifts in favor of behavior change. Finding such "teachable moments" when individuals are receptive to change and providing services quickly and easily are classic tactics of public health practice.

"Meeting people where they are" is a public health strategy that can be used to initiate low-threshold interventions.

1.3   Epidemiology

Development of a viable continuum of behavioral health services rests on understanding the population distribution and dynamics of behavioral health problems, patterns of care-seeking, and relationships between the two (Tucker, Phillips, Murphy, & Raczynski, 2004). The relevant behavioral epidemiology findings are summarized next.

1.3.1   Behavioral Health Problems in the General Population

Worldwide, MH/SU disorders contribute substantially to the global burden of disease and disability, and the great majority of persons with problems do not receive treatment (Wang et al., 2005; WHO World Mental Health Survey Consortium, 2004). About a third of the population experiences one or more diagnosable disorders on a lifetime basis, and many others experience subclinical signs and symptoms that may develop further or remit on their own. Mood disorders, including anxiety and depressive disorders, and alcohol and other substance use disorders are among the most prevalent disorders and contribute significantly to the global burden of disease and disability. Schizophrenia and other psychotic disorders, while much less common ($< 3\%$), also contribute significantly (US Surgeon General, 1999; WHO World Mental Health Survey Consortium, 2004).

Mood disorders and substance use disorders are highly prevalent, and most persons with these problems do not receive treatment.

1.3.2   Behavioral Health Problems in Medical Patients

Many medical patients have behavioral health problems such as depressive or substance use disorders (SUDs), or they engage in behavior patterns that adversely affect their health status, medical treatment adherence, and outcomes (Tucker et al., 2004). People who seek help for psychological symptoms often ask their primary care providers for help first, and the main complaint of many primary care patients has a psychological or behavioral component. The "worried well" are common in medical settings. Their problems may benefit from brief interventions or resolve without treatment. Some medical patients, however, will have more serious problems and will need more intensive evaluation, referral, and treatment.

Medical patients with psychological concerns are common, and many need help with medication adherence or lifestyle changes.

Behavioral health problems can be difficult to detect because medical patients often do not self-identify as having such problems; their problems often are fairly mild and do not meet diagnostic criteria; and busy primary care providers may not screen for them effectively (Pini, Perkonnig, Tansella, & Wittchen, 1999). Uncomplicated depressive, anxiety, and alcohol-related problems are most common and can be treated in medical settings. Most people who receive an intervention for depression are treated by primary care physicians, who write the majority of prescriptions for antidepressant medications (Lieberman, 2003). Treating depression is important because it is comorbid with many medical disorders and often contributes to poor medical outcomes.

Uncomplicated mood and substance use disorders can be treated with brief interventions in primary medical care settings.

As another example, SBIs for alcohol problems are recommended in primary care and emergency departments because such problems are prevalent among their patients. See http://pubs.niaaa.nih.gov/publications/Practitioner/CliniciansGuide2005/clinicians_guide.htm for an example of an evidence-based SBI recommended by the National Institute on Alcohol Abuse and Alcoholism (NIAAA, 2005).

1.3.3   Economic Impact

Reduced medical costs may offset costs of behavioral health treatments, but behavioral health benefits are often the first to be cut by third-party payers.

Behavioral health problems, especially when untreated, pose a substantial economic burden on the health care system and broader economy (US Surgeon General, 1999). Including behavioral health services in primary care and covering them in comprehensive health plans reduces the use and cost of medical services (Cummings, O'Donohue, & Ferguson, 2002). This *medical cost offset effect* provides an economic basis for covering behavioral health services in MCOs and other health plans and provider organizations. Despite the cost savings, however, behavioral health services are often among the first to be cut in cost-containment efforts, particularly before federal parity legislation was enacted.

1.4   Course and Prognosis

MH/SU disorders typically emerge in adolescence and early adulthood before age 25, and subthreshold symptoms often predate full clinical diagnosis (WHO World Mental Health Survey Consortium, 2004). Early adulthood is an important period for early case-finding and preventive interventions, in addition to treatment when indicated. Some disorders (e.g., SUDs) remit in many cases without treatment, particularly in early adulthood, whereas other disorders that occur early in life presage increased risk for future recurrences (e.g., schizophrenia, major depression).

Mental health and substance use disorders often emerge during adolescence and young adulthood. Many resolve without treatment or with brief intervention only.

For many MH/SU problems, partial or full improvement to premorbid levels of functioning occurs without treatment or with brief interventions. In some cases, improvements are sustained; in others, the risk of relapse remains high. The informed behavioral health practitioner will understand how population segments differ in the distribution and severity of MH/SU problems and the range of variations in the long-term course and need for continued monitoring with linkages to care.

Depression illustrates relationships between subthreshold and clinical presentations of disorders and how this can inform screening and practice patterns (Tucker et al., 2004). In the general US adult population, 20% to 30% of individuals experience subthreshold depressive symptoms, which may remit without intervention. However, only a minority of depressed individuals seek treatment, and even fewer receive specialty mental health care (Wang et al., 2005). Major depression, the most severe form of the disorder, occurs in less than 10% of cases, but it tends to recur; 50% of persons who have had one major depressive episode will have another, and 70% who have had two episodes will have a third. Thus, long-term monitoring of individuals with a history of major depression is a high priority in behavioral health care.

20% to 30% of the general US adult population have subthreshold depressive symptoms.

Relapse of major depression is common, and long-term monitoring is a high priority.

1.5 Differential Diagnosis

As discussed in Chapter 3, formal clinical diagnosis is not highly relevant to public health or integrated behavioral health practice. Rapid, macroscopic determination of whether care is needed, and if so the appropriate level of care, is more central to practice. This is the case because the focus of public health and integrated behavioral health care often is on the large untreated population segment with risk factors or subclinical forms of disorders. This untreated segment tends to have less severe problems than clinical samples, and they often fall short of fulfilling all diagnostic criteria.

Behavioral health assessment is more concerned with rapid, macroscopic determinations about need for care than with formal clinical diagnosis.

1.6 Comorbidities

Comorbid conditions are common among persons with MH/SU disorders. For example, more than 20% of people with a mental disorder in the United States also have a substance use disorder (Wang et al., 2005). Persons with comorbidities generally need specialty clinical care that falls outside the services discussed in this book.

Comorbid MH/SU conditions are common and typically require specialty clinical care.

1.7 Diagnostic Procedures and Documentation

The psychological and behavioral problems of individuals need to be considered in an integrated behavioral health model of practice, and practitioners need to be competent with established assessment procedures and diagnostic systems. However, as discussed in Chapter 3, the scope of assessment is generally broader than the focus of traditional clinical assessment and diagnosis on individual characteristics. In an expanded population approach to practice, primary objectives of assessment are to identify opportunities for intervention delivery to persons who do not present for treatment and to characterize their motivations for change and determine where they are in the change process.

Identifying and exploiting opportunities to be of service is central to the behavioral health approach.

Finding and exploiting these opportunities within systems and communities, as well as at the individual level, is a new domain of assessment for mental health practitioners. Consumer preferences and needs should guide the development and delivery of behavioral health programs. The scope of assessment should be multileveled and cover service features that matter to end-point consumers, such as provider characteristics, privacy, and cost, as well as features of the health care system that can promote appropriate service utilization, such as convenient parking and appointments with minimal waiting times. Another assessment objective in some applications is to screen and triage clients quickly to appropriate services that range from brief interventions to outpatient or inpatient treatment.

After describing theories that have guided public health and integrated behavioral health care in Chapter 2, these alternative assessment goals and methods are discussed in Chapter 3. Evidence-based public health and behavioral health interventions for MH/SU disorders that involve varying degrees of individualization and often make use of phone and computer technologies to extend the reach of care are then described in Chapter 4. A case vignette presented in Chapter 5 illustrates how several services along the continuum of care from low to high threshold and intensity can be applied to the medical and behavioral health care of persons living with HIV/AIDS.

2

Theories and Models of Behavior Change in Behavioral Health Practice

Psychology's unique role in public health is to act as the steward of a correct application of behavioral knowledge and theory.
Laura C. Leviton, *American Psychologist,* 1996

Psychologists have been in the vanguard of developing theoretical approaches to understanding individual differences in health behavior, and these theories and models have been widely applied to health promotion and preventive care (Glanz, Rimer, & Viswanath, 2008). Broadly defined, theory is a systematic relationship of constructs that are devised to analyze, predict, and explain the nature of a specified set of phenomena under a relatively wide variety of circumstances. A theory must be empirically testable and generalizable across settings and populations. According to McGuire (1983), the adequacy of a theory can be assessed in terms of three criteria: (1) its logic or internal consistency, (2) the extent to which it is parsimonious and broadly relevant while using a manageable number of constructs, and (3) its plausibility (e.g., does it fit with prevailing concepts and data in the field?). At its best, a theory guides both research and application, and directs attention toward relationships that can be evaluated empirically. Findings then support refinements of concepts, hypotheses, and applications.

> Theory should be internally consistent, parsimonious, and plausible and guide both research and practice.

The variable domains relevant to health behavior change and public health practice span intrapersonal, interpersonal, and broader contextual variables reflecting community, economic, organizational, and policy levels (Glanz et al., 2008; National Cancer Institute [NCI], 2003). At the intrapersonal level, theories focus on factors within an individual such as attitudes, motivation, knowledge, and skills, whereas interpersonal theories postulate that other people in one's social network influence behavior. Theories emphasizing the individual as the unit of analysis are common in psychology, and we refer to them as *psychological theories* (regardless of the disciplinary origin). In contrast, *contextual theories* are broader in scope and seek to explain individual and group behavior in context. They focus on how behavior is affected by factors such as social norms, community, and ecological characteristics; economic variables; health system characteristics; and public policy (NCI, 2003). These theories tend to be multilevel with respect to units of analysis and are more common in sociology, economics, and ecology.

> Psychological theories focus on intrapersonal and interpersonal factors. Contextual theories seek to explain behavior in a broader environmental context.

Theories can vary along several additional dimensions, including: (1) the extent to which they are primarily explanatory and concerned with illuminating the nature of a given phenomenon or problem, or are useful for directing the development and implementation of behavior change interventions (Green,

2000); (2) whether they are predominately inductive or deductive in nature, which reflects the degree to which empirical findings precede or follow theoretical development, respectively; and (3) the extent to which the dimension of time is incorporated in concepts and applications. The first two dimensions are not rigid distinctions; e.g., some theories provide both explanation and application regarding behavior change. However, whether a theory deals with time is a clear-cut distinction that is basic to understanding the temporal dynamics of behavior change and influencing its course in positive ways. Absent concern with time, a theory can inform structural or static variables that are associated with behavior patterns and outcomes at a given point in time, but will be limited with respect to predicting and controlling trajectories of behavior through time, which is the essence of behavior change. Holding time constant is sometimes necessary to conceptualize and measure complex systems (e.g., health care systems), but complexity should not be confused with explanation of behavior change. The psychological and contextual theories discussed in this chapter vary considerably in their specifics, and each has made important contributions in the health arena. However, these more basic dimensions of theoretical construction should be kept in mind because they often determine the utility of a theory for informing practice in real world settings more than the theoretical specifics. We return to these issues after presenting the different theories.

> Incorporating the temporal dimension of behavior over time is critical for a theory to guide behavior change applications effectively.

2.1   Psychological Theories

Table 2 summarizes the major features of four psychological theories relevant to public health, including two intrapersonal theories (health belief model [HBM] and theory of reasoned action/theory of planned behavior [TRA/TPB]), an interpersonal theory (social cognitive theory [SCT]), and a theory that combines elements of both (transtheoretical model [TTM]). The first three are expectancy-value theories, which hold that behavior is determined by the value placed on a particular outcome and by one's estimate of the likelihood that a given behavior will result in that outcome. The TTM recognizes expectancy-value constructs, such as weighing the pros and cons of change, and incorporates constructs from a variety of theories. However, it is primarily a cross-cutting framework that describes the steps and processes of behavior change over time, not causal relationships (Glanz et al., 2008).

> Expectancy is the belief that a behavior will produce a desired outcome. Value is the importance placed on the outcome.

2.1.1   Expectancy-Value Theories

The HBM is one of the oldest and most recognized interpersonal theories (e.g., Rosenstock, 1974) and was developed to help explain why few people took advantage of screening services for tuberculosis. It has since been widely applied as a model of utilization of other health screening and intervention programs (e.g., mammography, cervical cancer screening, high blood pressure, and adherence behaviors). Initially, the model had five constructs: (1) *perceived susceptibility* to a health risk; (2) *perceived severity* of a health problem; (3) *perceived benefits* (or positive consequences) of, and; (4) *perceived*

Table 2
Psychological Theories

Health belief model
- Perceived susceptibility (risk of experiencing the condition)
- Perceived severity (consequences or outcomes) of the condition
- Perceived benefits of adopting behavior
- Perceived barriers or disadvantages to adopting behavior
- Cues to action (internal or external events that influence decision-making)

Theory of reasoned action/Theory of planned behavior
- Behavioral beliefs and evaluation → attitude toward behavior
- Normative beliefs and motivation to comply → subjective norms about behavior
- Control beliefs and perceived power → perceived behavioral control (TPB only)
- Attitudes, subjective norms, perceived control → behavioral intentions
- All behavior is the result of intentions

Social cognitive theory
- Reciprocal determinism (interaction of person, behavior, and environment)
- Behavioral capability (skills to do behavior)
- Outcome expectancies (belief that behavior will produce desired results)
- Self-efficacy (confidence to perform a specific behavior when needed)
- Observational learning (watching behaviors and outcomes of others)
- Reinforcements (consequences of behavior that promote continued change)

Transtheoretical model
- Stages of change (different degrees of readiness to change)
- Processes of change (cognitive or behavioral)
- Decisional balance (weighing pros and cons of change)
- Self-efficacy (confidence to perform a specific behavior when needed)

Note. TPB = Theory of planned behavior

barriers to (or negative consequences of) avoiding the health problem; and (5) *cues to action* that may influence decisions to act (e.g., physical symptoms, mass media messages). *Perceived self-efficacy* was later added to the model, which is the strength of belief in one's ability to carry out a given behavior successfully (Bandura, 1977). Successful interventions are those that increase perceived benefits of change, while minimizing perceived and actual barriers to change. The HBM was important for directing attention toward the study of delays in care-seeking. However, it does not have strong power to predict change and is less efficacious with more complex behaviors (Harrison, Mullen, & Green, 1992).

According to the original TRA (Fishbein & Ajzen, 1975) and its modification, the TPB (Ajzen, 1985), an individual's attitudes, normative beliefs (perception of peers' attitudes), and the desire to comply with peers to obtain their approval all interact to a form a "behavioral intention" to act in a specific way. All behavior is considered to result from such intentions, which are a cognitive representation of one's readiness to perform a behavior. Intentions are immediate antecedents of behavior and reflect the likelihood of performing the behavior.

Interventions guided by the health belief model try to increase perceived benefits of change and decrease perceived and actual barriers.

The theory of reasoned action/ planned behavior is a cognitive model. Intent is viewed as the immediate antecedent and determinant of behavior.

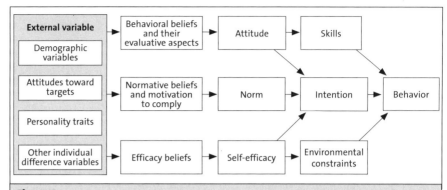

Figure 3
Social cognitive theory. Figure depicts one hypothesized model of how social cognitive constructs lead to behavior change. Adapted from *Theory at a Glance: A Guide for Health Promotion Practice* (2nd ed.), by National Cancer Institute, 2003, Bethesda, MD: US Department of Health and Human Services.

Ajzen (1985) added the construct of *perceived control* to account for situations in which people held the intention to engage in a behavior but did not do so. The greater the perceived control over factors such as behavioral opportunities, resources, and skills, and the more favorable the attitude and subjective norms, the stronger a person's intention to perform a given behavior should be. The addition of the perceived control construct helped explain relationships between intention and actual behavior, and the recognition that behavioral intention cannot be the exclusive determinant of behavior was a major contribution of the TRA/TPB.

Social learning theory (Bandura, 1977) and its later outgrowth SCT (Bandura, 1986) proposed that behavior is the result of continuous interactions among the person, his or her behaviors, and the environment. A change in one component presumably affects the others via a process of *reciprocal determinism*. SCT further proposed that reinforcement of a behavior leads to expectations about outcomes (*outcome expectancies*) and the effect of behavior on outcomes (*response efficacy*). Figure 3 outlines SCT constructs and methods that can be used to encourage adoption of health-promoting behaviors.

> Reciprocal determinism is the synergistic interaction of individual, behavior, and environment.

In expanding and renaming his theory SCT, Bandura (1986) asserted that self-efficacy is the major construct underlying many aspects of behavior change. If people are confident about their ability to make a change (e.g., taking medication on schedule), they will do so even when faced with adversities. However, if people have low confidence in their ability to make a change, there is little motivation to act, and if they do act, they will not persist when faced with even minimal resistance.

2.1.2 Transtheoretical Model of Change

> The transtheoretical model addresses the processes of behavior change across different systems of psychotherapy, more so than determinants of change.

Prochaska and DiClemente (e.g., Prochaska & DiClemente, 1984) developed the TTM (also known as the "stages-of-change model") to describe and explain behavior change processes that were common across different systems of psychotherapy and therefore were "transthereotical." The model expanded the scope of inquiry beyond therapy-assisted change to include self-change

Techniques to Promote Change in Each Stage of the Transtheoretical Model

(1) *Precontemplation:* People in the precontemplation stage need to become more aware of the benefits of change, e.g., through consciousness-raising activities such as behavioral monitoring or thinking about reasons why they engage in a problem behavior.

(2) *Contemplation:* People in the contemplation stage are ambivalent. Useful techniques at this stage include reevaluating the impact of one's behavior on others or clarifying personal values and self-identify and how one's behavior does or does not fit with them.

(3) *Preparation:* The preparation stage comprises both an intention and a behavioral criterion that is not yet consistently performed. For example, a sexually active man may intend to use condoms every time he has sex, but he does so inconsistently or without positive results (e.g., the condom breaks). In addition to skill-building, people in the preparation stage can benefit from action prompts such as posting notes as reminders; avoiding people, places, and objects associated with unhealthy behavior patterns; and developing contingency plans.

(4) *Action:* This stage entails behavior that meets accepted action criteria for a given health behavior; e.g., the action criterion for smoking cessation is zero cigarettes smoked, not even a puff. Social support, rewarding oneself for taking action, and avoiding relapse are hallmarks of the action stage, which for many behaviors lasts up to 6 months.

(5) *Maintenance:* Individuals in the maintenance stage are attempting to sustain change over time and need to continue developing alternate ways of dealing with high risk situations. Some successful changers will become advocates of change for others, which helps them to maintain their success. However, relapse or regression to an earlier stage can occur at any time in the change process. Slipping back into unhealthy behavior patterns, at least for a time, is expected. Such efforts should not be considered failures because many people resume positive change after a slip or lapse (Grimley, Prochaska, & Prochaska, 1997). With smoking, for example, it takes the average smoker three or four serious quit attempts before cessation is reliably maintained.

and other processes that occur before and after time-limited treatments. The theory rapidly took root in research on smoking cessation, which often occurs via self-change, and it has since been applied widely to the cessation or adoption of a broad range of behaviors.

Four major constructs make up the TTM: the stages of change, the processes of change, decisional balance, and perceived self-efficacy (e.g., Prochaska, DiClemente, & Norcross, 1992). The TTM postulates that when modifying behaviors, individuals cycle through five stages of change. The text box describes each stage and gives examples of change techniques that are relevant to promoting change in each stage.

The techniques used in the different stages represent some of the processes of change, another construct of the TTM. For most behaviors, 10 processes of change have been identified, five of which are cognitive or affective (e.g., self-evaluation, consciousness raising) and five of which are behavioral (e.g., contingency management, helping relations). The processes of change are covert and overt activities hypothesized to facilitate progression though the stages (Prochaska et al., 1992). Additional constructs include decisional bal-

---

Do you smoke?
- No → behavior not relevant
- Yes ↓

1. Are you seriously thinking about quitting in the next 6 months?
- No → precontemplation
- Yes ↓

2. Are you seriously thinking about quitting in the next 30 days?
- No → contemplation
- Yes ↓

3. Have you made at least one serious quit attempt in the last year?
- No → contemplation
- Yes → preparation

Figure 4
How to determine a person's stage of change for smoking cessation

---

ance (weighing the pros and cons of changing) and self-efficacy. The basic intervention approach that follows from the TTM is to individualize intervention messages and strategies based on assessment of an individual's current stage of readiness for change. Figure 4 shows how an individual smoker's stage of change for smoking cessation can be assessed.

The TTM has had great heuristic value in understanding the behavior change process and in shifting attention to variables other than treatment-specific characteristics. However, it has been criticized on several grounds. A major criticism is the lack of continued exploration of more powerful predictors (constructs) that could potentially expand the model's usefulness when applied to more diverse and complex behaviors. Similar to other intrapersonal theories, the TTM also lacks much focus on contextual, structural, or historical factors that may affect behavior. However, it differs from the other psychological theories in its explicit focus on trajectories of change, which is a major strength. Empirical support for the TTM has been mixed; e.g., the supporting evidence is weak for distinct stages, progression through the stages, and hypothesized relationships between the stages and processes; different measures of readiness to change have yielded discrepant stage assignments; and behavioral outcomes have not been consistently related to progression through the stages (Joseph, Breslin, & Skinner, 1999; Napper et al., 2008).

Despite these limitations, the TTM has made enduring contributions to health promotion. These include its expansion of the scope of and temporal perspective on behavior change, the emphasis it places on characterizing readiness and motivation for change, and its provision of a basis for intervention matching.

2.2   Contextual Theories

The main features of two prominent contextual models, the social-ecological (SE) and behavioral economics (BE) models, are presented in Table 3 and discussed next.

Table 3
Contextual Models

Social-ecological model
- Not so much a theory as an overarching perspective
- Five levels of influence on behavior
  - Intrapersonal
  - Interpersonal
  - Institutional
  - Community
  - Public policy
- Levels interact and are interdependent
- Multiple factors emanating from all five levels influence behavior
- Multilevel interventions encouraged (e.g., antismoking media campaign combined with restrictions on public smoking and sales to minors)

Behavioral economics
- Choice is the distribution of behavior to available activities and commodities over time
- Contextual factors influence behavioral allocation
- Reward amount and temporal availability (delay to reward receipt) influence choice
- People tend to prefer a larger later reward until access to a smaller sooner reward is imminent
- People devalue delayed rewards at different "discount" rates
- Can be used to study health states and outcomes, behaviors, and service utilization

2.2.1   Social-Ecological Model

The IOM (2003) has suggested that the multilevel perspective offered by the SE model may be essential to bringing about improvements in population health. The Institute asserted that an understanding of the determinants of health from a multilevel ecological perspective is necessary to develop, implement, and evaluate effective interventions to enhance public health. Multilevel interventions have potential for synergies of effective interventions across various levels, which could facilitate and sustain positive health-related outcomes. In reality, however, such multilevel intervention approaches are rare, perhaps because the ecological perspective is *too* comprehensive. Because of their complexity, ecological models have not yielded guidelines or principles for health promotion (Edberg, 2009).

The social-ecological model encourages intervention at multiple levels of the environment.

Figure 5 provides one example of a social-ecological model (IOM, 2003). The word *ecology* originates in the biological sciences and refers to the interrelationships between organisms and their environments. In public health and the social and behavioral sciences, an ecological model examines how the social environment – consisting of intrapersonal, interpersonal, organizational, community, and public policy levels – supports and maintains risk behaviors. These five levels of influence determine health and well-being, and each level is a potential target for health promotion intervention (Glantz, Rimer, Viswanath, 2008).

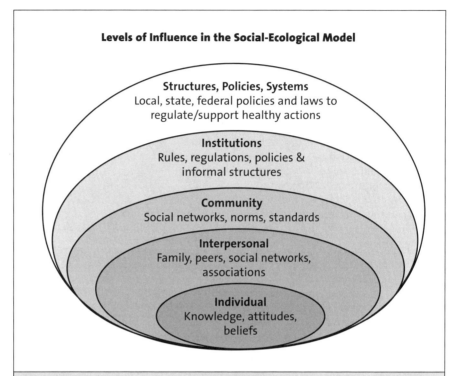

Figure 5
Social-ecological perspective. This figure shows multiple determinants of population health and well-being that are related and linked. Adapted from *Who Will Keep the Public Healthy? Educating Public Health Professionals for the 21st Century,* by the Institute of Medicine, 2003, Washington, DC: National Academies Press.

2.2.2   Behavioral Economics

BE is another contextual theory with a strong empirical base. This transdisciplinary framework has roots in operant psychology and consumer demand theory in microeconomics and is useful for understanding the role of the environment in behavioral choice (e.g., Ainslie, 1975; Bickel & Vuchinich, 2003). Choice is viewed as how behavior is distributed to available activities and commodities over time, not as a cognitive process. BE focuses on how features of the context of choice influence behavioral allocation patterns (e.g., time, money, or effort). A robust generalization is that preference for a given activity or commodity is context dependent, and its value can be inferred from the relative resources allocated to obtain it.

Preferences change over time depending on the availability of, and constraints on, the activities in the context of choice. BE focuses on dynamic "now versus later" relationships between choices that involve different commodities that vary in value and delay to receipt (Ainslie, 1975). Research on such "intertemporal" choice has shown that delayed rewards are devalued or "discounted" in an orderly way that can be described mathematically by hyperbolic discount functions. As shown in Figure 6, the perceived immediate value of a given alternative rises sharply immediately before the opportunity

> **In behavioral economics, choice is the distribution of behavior. It is not a cognitive process.**

> **Delay to receipt of a reward influences its perceived value. Delayed rewards are generally devalued or "discounted."**

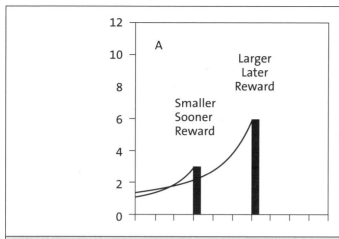

Figure 6
Temporal dynamics of behavioral choice. Graph shows an intertemporal choice between a smaller sooner reward (SSR) and a larger later reward (LLR). The area under the curve is the value of each reward at a given point in time based on hyperbolic discounting of future rewards. The LLR will be preferred until the availability of the SSR becomes imminent, at which point an abrupt preference reversal in favor of the SSR occurs. Adapted from "Specious Reward: A Behavioral Theory of Impulsiveness and Impulse Control," by G. Ainslie, 1975, *Psychological Bulletin, 82*, 463–509.

for its receipt. Research has also shown that people differ in the rates at which they discount delayed rewards. For instance, children exhibit higher discount rates than adults, and persons with addictive disorders exhibit higher rates than nonaddicted adults. Nevertheless, a highly valued delayed reward, or series of such later larger rewards (LLR), will be preferred over a smaller sooner reward (SSR), as long as the choice is made before the availability of the SSR is imminent. Then, there often is a preference reversal in favor of the SSR. Preference usually reverts back to the LLR when the availability of the SSR passes, as long as the LLR remains available.

BE has been applied widely to investigate health states and outcomes, health protective and risk behaviors, and health services utilization (e.g., Bickel & Vuchinich, 2003; Tucker, Simpson, & Khodneva, 2010b). Many health behaviors involve intertemporal trade-offs between choices for future positive health outcomes versus more immediately rewarding, less prohealth behavior. For example, unhealthy but enjoyable eating habits are experienced by many people as a choice between immediate rewards with longer-term costs. In contrast, a pattern of healthy eating and exercise is experienced as less rewarding short-term, but valuable for longer-term health and the positive opportunities that good health allows.

> Health behaviors may involve trade-offs between smaller sooner rewards and later larger rewards.

Although such real-world trade-offs in health choices are typically diffuse and occur as a series of many choices over a long time, individuals are able to contemplate directly the trade-off of future health (or future life-expectancy) for the immediate receipt of desirable non-health goods and commodities (Tucker et al., 2010b). For example, in a seminal study (Chapman & Johnson, 1995), healthy young adults evaluated choices between hypothetical amounts of reduced life-expectancy (in days to years) and valuable non-health com-

> Choice biases can be incorporated into health-promotion strategies.

Alternative Strategies for Behavior Change: Remediating Choice Biases or Manipulating the Architecture of Choice

Given that individuals discount health outcomes and make short-term choices that often are not beneficial longer term, behavioral economics (BE) directs attention to two intervention strategies that have received some support in behavior change research (Tucker et al., 2010b): (1) attempt to remediate the choice biases of decision-makers (e.g., through self-control training or similar strategies) or provide incentives for better choices (e.g., through environmental restructuring or awarding voucher incentives for desirable behaviors) (Bickel & Marsch, 2000); or (2) accept that biased choices are the norm, and structure health messages, choices, interventions, and contexts in ways that use the biases to promote good choices and health outcomes (Loewenstein, Brennan, & Volpp, 2007).

Psychotherapeutic approaches tend to emphasize the former remedial strategy, whereas BE and public health approaches make more use of the latter "architecture of choice" strategy. An example of the first strategy would be to teach individuals to view their choices as patterns of behavior with different longer term costs and benefits in order to increase choice of health options that yield the best overall benefit (Rachlin, 1995).

An example of the second strategy that incorporates choice biases to promote health is illustrated by the *asymmetrical paternalism* strategy for improving health behaviors developed by Loewenstein et al. (2007). As a prototypic example involving discounting of long-term benefits of healthy food choices, they recommended changing the order of food presentation in a cafeteria line so that healthy foods are presented before desserts. The overall availability of desserts is unchanged, but the switch helps overweight or hungry people with suboptimal self-control make better food choices. The strategy exploits choice biases (delay discounting in this case) to help those most susceptible to them make better choices without otherwise infringing on freedom of choice. The two approaches are not mutually exclusive, and research is needed to determine what mix of options works best.

modities to be received immediately. Participants were willing to swap days and weeks of their life for durable goods such as televisions or cars and for immediately consumable goods including beer and snacks. The text box shows how these common choice biases can be approached therapeutically for purposes of promoting sound choices and positive behavior change.

BE has strong empirical support in research that spans basic experiments on choice with animals and humans, clinical interventions for addictive and other health behaviors, and policies concerned with national drug control and improving personal savings rates (Madden & Bickel, 2010; Tucker & Simpson, in press). Among behavior change theories, BE has the most explicit and well-developed analysis of the temporal dynamics of change. Another strength is that BE provides common concepts and terms that can be used across multiple disciplines, as is often needed in effective public health and policy applications. A criticism of the approach is that it is not "psychological" enough and runs counter to common notions about the causes of human behavior that put the controlling variables inside the person or in the immediate antecedent conditions preceding behavior. BE is a "molar" perspective that seeks to account for regularities between environmental contexts and behavior patterns over time. Unlike many psychological theories, it does not focus on discrete, temporally contiguous environment–behavior relationships.

Behavioral economics stresses contexts and patterns of behavior over time.

2.3   Health Communication

Communication theory is a field unto itself, comprising models of information processing, such as from cognitive psychology, and descriptive models that explain how information diffuses through a community or culture. Although detailed explication of the field is beyond the scope of this book, the behavioral health "tool box" is not complete without communication frameworks and strategies that support the population focus of public health. Many theories described in this chapter have been used successfully to guide development of health promotion messages for individuals, but a carefully crafted message is of little use if it is not disseminated successfully to the public. Conversely, a framework of how to disseminate information addresses only the means and methods of communication, not the content.

Both the content and process of a health promotion activity must be sound for an intervention to succeed.

Constructs and determinants from the psychological and contextual theories presented earlier must be employed to create meaningful content that promotes healthful behaviors. More fundamentally, carefully crafted content that is communicated well cannot compensate for environmental constraints such as limited access to health care, restricted availability of health-promoting activities, or policy failures to address such needs (NCI, 2001). Despite these caveats, development, dissemination and evaluation of health-promoting messages is a critical component of behavioral health care. Table 4 summarizes three major communication models, which are discussed next.

McGuire (1984) proposed an information processing model (IPM) that describes steps through which an individual must pass to adopt a behavior: exposure, perception, comprehension, agreement, retention, retrieval, decision-making, and action. As outlined in Table 4, these may be evaluated through a series of five questions. To ensure that these questions are answered in the affirmative, five components of communication must be implemented successfully (NCI, 2001). The IPM is a useful framework for assuring that the process of communicating content helps, rather than hinders, behavior change.

Information processing addresses the steps required to persuade an audience.

The diffusion of innovations model (DOI; Rogers, 2003) is another useful theory that helps explain how new behaviors become established in communities. Diffusion is a process by which an innovation is communicated through certain channels over time among members of a group or population. An innovation can be a new idea, product, or social practice. The adoption of an innovation depends on some combination of well-established personal ties (word of mouth) and mass media. Communication is viewed as a "two-step flow process" in which "opinion leaders" in the community mediate the effects of mass media communications. Therefore, emphasis is placed on the significance of social networks, above and beyond mass media, to persuade people to adopt an innovation (NCI, 2003).

Diffusion of innovation describes how a new idea or behavior moves into the mainstream community.

When planning a health promotion campaign, training and mobilizing the support of opinion leaders can greatly increase the chances that an innovation will be adopted in a community. Because they are trusted, opinion leaders have credibility to communicate five key pieces of information about the behavior change being promoted, as summarized in Table 4 (NCI, 2003).

According to the DOI model, new innovations are effectively diffused when a critical mass of opinion leaders (innovators and early adopters), usually 16% of the total target population, adopt the innovation (Oldenberg & Glanz, 2008).

Table 4
Communication Theories

Information processing model
- Did the individual pay attention to the message?
- Comprehend it?
- Believe it?
- Remember it?
- Behave accordingly?
- Five components must be addressed to ensure successful processing:
  - Source credibility
  - Message design
  - Delivery channel
  - Intended audience
  - Intended behavior

Diffusion of innovations
- New ideas (innovations) are communicated through channels to diffuse through a social system over time.
- Relative advantage: Is the innovation superior to existing options?
- Compatibility: Does it fit with audience values, lifestyle, and so on?
- Complexity: Is it simple to use or understand?
- Trialability: Can people "try before they buy"?
- Observability: Can adopters easily see and measure results?
- Two-step flow of communications: Media → opinion leaders → other community members

Social marketing
- Market segmentation: targeting specific subpopulations rather than using generic messages
- Product (desired behavior)
- Price (time, effort, social effects as well as money)
- Place (communication channel: e.g., TV versus print)
- Promotion (selling behavior as one would sell a consumer product)

Figure 7 illustrates the postulated bell curve of diffusion. By sharing information, delivering intervention messages, endorsing the innovation, and modeling effective methods of behavior change, opinion leaders help change social norms and facilitate change in the behavior of those in the community (NCI, 2003).

Social marketing is a third consumer-focused approach that takes communication techniques with demonstrated effectiveness in the commercial business sector and uses them to improve public health (Weinreich, 1999). These commercial techniques use the "marketing mix" of product, price, place, and promotion in service of advancing social causes. Marketing focuses on consumers and is aimed at identifying the needs and wants of specific subgroups in the population. A core principle in social marketing is *market segmentation*, which is the practice of identifying distinct groups in the population to which specific products, services, or messages are to be directed. Groups may be variously based on demographics (e.g., age, gender), health or MH/SU status (e.g., problems such as depression or heavy drinking), geographic location or dispersion, race or ethnicity, and values (e.g., independence, fairness, rebellion, or control). Targeting allows practitioners to select appropriate

Market segmentation is the key to social marketing success.

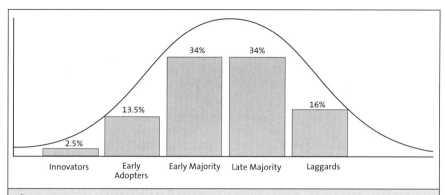

Figure 7
Diffusion of Innovations theory. Bell curve shows how new ideas (innovations) are communicated through channels to diffuse through a social system over time and how different population subgroups tend to adopt innovations at different points in the diffusion process (Based on Rogers, 2003).

messages, sources (e.g., spokespersons), and delivery channels for each audience segment (Weinreich, 1999). Qualitative and quantitative data collection are typically used with a subgroup of the target segment to gain an in-depth understanding of what reaches and motivates them (see Chapter 3). As Figure 8 illustrates, this is an iterative process. Data are gathered continuously until the final product has appeal and value to the target audience (NCI, 2001).

This approach deserves greater application and evaluation, and its consumer-centric orientation is compatible with other theories of health decision-making, such as behavioral economics, and other theories of behavior change. However, research is very limited, and outcome evaluations comparing a social marketing product or program with a conventionally developed health promotion program are lacking (Grier & Bryant, 2005).

All of the communication theories are persuasive in nature, but some caveats regarding their application to health communication are in order. A meta-analysis by Witte and Allen (2000) found that behavior change is most likely when fear and efficacy appeals are combined. When efficacy messaging is limited or not addressed, however, fear appeals are more likely to result in message avoidance. Smokers, for example, may "tune out" a health campaign message that stokes fear of lung cancer unless confidence to quit also is bolstered. Finally, persuasive techniques may strike a negative chord with the public due to their association with corporate and political messaging, and care should be taken to avoid actual or apparent coercion or manipulation of facts when these methods are used to disseminate health messages (Guttman, 2003).

2.4   Theoretical Themes and Implications for Behavioral Health Change

Despite many specific differences in the theoretical perspectives, several themes emerge across theories about the essential nature of health behavior change and the variable domains that warrant consideration in planning

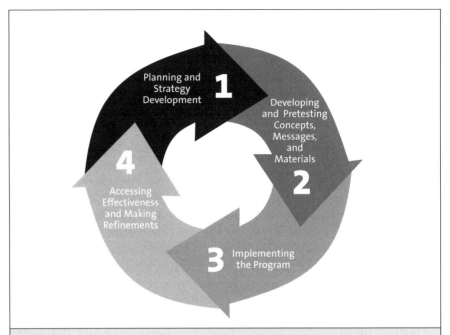

Figure 8
Social marketing wheel. Framework emphasizes formative research and evaluation, as well as outcome evaluation. Three of four stages focus on planning and modification, rather than implementation. Adapted from *Theory at a Glance: A Guide for Health Promotion Practice* (2nd ed.), by National Cancer Institute, 2003, Bethesda, MD: US Department of Health and Human Services.

Individuals change in context, change occurs over time, and psychological and contextual variables both influence the change process.

assessments and interventions to promote change. Fundamentally, individuals change in context, and the change process occurs over time. Individual characteristics matter, but so does the broader context, and a comprehensive understanding will require concern with both psychological and contextual variables over time.

For example, within the psychological realm, influential variables include an individual's motivation for and readiness to change, personal resources, self-efficacy expectations about executing behaviors required for change, and habitual decision-making style (e.g., impulsivity and heavy discounting of future outcomes). With regard to context, the social network can be quite influential on health-seeking behaviors in both positive and negative ways, and some problems require intervening with networks as well as individuals. Stigma, a fundamentally social phenomenon, remains a deterrent to care for several behavioral health disorders (e.g., SUDs), and persons with such problems may surface in nonspecialty medical settings.

The context of health care, such as location and waiting time, influences health-seeking behaviors.

Features of health care systems and economic factors also can deter or facilitate treatment entry. For example, rapid appointments on demand promote utilization, whereas long waiting times deter utilization (Tucker & Davison, 2000). Until the recent passage of federal parity legislation in the United States, greater restrictions on insurance benefits for outpatient MH/SU visits compared with equivalent medical care were a common barrier to adequate care. The US Patient Protection and Affordable Care Act of 2010 also reiterates parity requirements and expands mental health care access via Medicare and Medicaid (American Psychological Association, 2010). However, full implementation will not occur until 2014, by which time further legislation may expand or contract insurance reform.

As discussed in the next chapter, these kinds of individual and contextual variables merit consideration and assessment in behavior change programs. Although conventional clinical diagnoses are often relevant, they are insufficient for directing many public health and integrated behavioral health care endeavors. Additional assessment issues involve finding opportunities for community outreach, SBIs, assessing consumer needs and preferences, and assessing motivation and readiness for change and elements of the surrounding context that may promote or deter change. At the core, the overarching goal is to reach beyond high-threshold clinical care into risk groups and communities and to provide access to evidence-based professional resources that do not include being a psychotherapy client or otherwise entering the health care system.

3

Diagnosis and Treatment Indications

In a typical clinical interaction, a reasonably motivated client presents for treatment, and the clinician uses the established tools of psychological and behavioral assessment and formal diagnostic criteria to formulate a course of treatment, usually via outpatient psychotherapy. Ideally, treatment will continue until the client improves, and termination will be a mutual client–therapist decision. Even when coercive elements exist for treatment entry (e.g., legal or employment concerns), or clients are resistant or relatively unmotivated to

---

The Role of Clinical Diagnosis in Public and Integrated Behavioral Health Practice

Clinical diagnosis using formal classification systems has not been particularly useful for guiding practice outside of clinical care. This may change as the *Diagnostic and Statistical Manual of Mental Disorders* (DSM), published commercially by the American Psychiatric Association, and the *International Classification of Diseases* (ICD), published by the World Health Organization as a free resource for the global community, undergo their next major revisions due for release by 2015 (Martin, 2009). The ICD is widely used internationally, whereas the DSM is mainly used in the United States. This is changing as more psychologists treat medically ill patients for whom there are now health and behavior codes based on the ICD system (Reed et al., 2005). The US Health Insurance Portability and Accountability Act (HIPAA) of 1996 also requires providers to use ICD codes in electronic transactions (Martin, 2009).

Heretofore, the two diagnostic systems were similar as regards MH/SU disorders, but they are expected to diverge more in the next revisions: the DSM-V and the ICD-11. The need to broaden the base of MH/SU services in the direction of public health services, in order to reduce the population burden of these disorders, is a major impetus for the expected divergence (Martin, 2009). Prior revisions of both systems trended toward greater complexity and differentiation among larger and larger numbers of disorder categories, but this made it difficult to use the schemes in field settings when quick decisions were required, often from paraprofessionals, about the need for and level of services.

The ICD revision seeks to simplify its system in ways that increase utility in public health settings. The ICD revision is expected to have fewer and broader disorder categories, as well as simplified diagnostic criteria within categories (Martin, 2009). Preliminary indications are that the DSM revision will entail greater complexity, in part because a dimensional approach to diagnosis will likely supplement select diagnostic categories such as SUDs (Helzer et al., 2008). A more difficult diagnostic scheme that is hard to reconcile with the ICD system that physicians use may further complicate and marginalize opportunities for collaboration in health care settings. Psychologists interested in pursuing the practice opportunities discussed in this book should follow these developments.

participate and change, the same sequence tends to be followed, albeit often with less than optimal results.

As the text box discusses, clinical diagnostic systems often are not highly relevant in an integrated behavioral health model of practice. Rather, the primary goal of assessment in public health and integrated behavioral health care is to find opportunities for intervention delivery to persons who do not seek treatment and to characterize their motivations for change and where they may be in the change process. Another important objective is to screen and triage clients quickly to appropriate services that range from brief interventions to outpatient or inpatient treatment. This chapter discusses this expanded view of assessment, in which conventional diagnosis and assessment are only one of several dimensions to consider in intervention planning.

> **The usual goal of public health assessment is not to diagnose individuals with clinical conditions, but to identify intervention opportunities.**

3.1   Finding Opportunities for Intervention Delivery

Public health practice is often opportunistic and, at its best, prevention-oriented. Common methods include early case-finding and quarantine, vaccination when available, and health education. The goal is to reach as many people as possible in the at-risk population with an easily disseminated preventive intervention that can have a significant impact on population health. A recent example is making human papillomavirus (HPV) vaccination available to adolescent girls and young women to prevent several virus-induced forms of cervical cancer.

Although the typical mental health practitioner will not deliver services on a population-based scale, many levels and channels for intervention that go beyond psychological services for individual clients are within reach of clinicians. As discussed in Chapter 1, these include services in the indicated and selective prevention sectors, early case-finding, and long-term extensive monitoring and stepped care for chronic conditions (see Figure 1). Familiar examples of preventive services include contributing behavioral expertise to wellness programs in hospitals and other large organizations. Such programs often yield *cost-offset benefits* for group health plans and organizations that pay for the wellness program, at least in part (Cummings et al., 2002). Other assessment and intervention opportunities involve using the vast amount of time that patients spend waiting for routine health care (Tucker & Davison, 2000). Waiting time can be put to good use for health-relevant assessment, education, and intervention. And the rapidly growing population adoption of cell phone and computer technology means that the possibilities for *telehealth* applications as an adjunct to or substitute for clinical care are nearly limitless.

> **Psychologists may expand their practices through indicated and selective prevention, case finding, long-term monitoring, and stepped care.**

Finding and exploiting these opportunities within organizations and communities is a new practice domain for many mental health practitioners. In today's health care market place, successful practitioners will not limit their practices to self-referred psychotherapy clients, but will look for new ways to extend the venues and reach of services to at-risk groups that are not seeking treatment. This chapter discusses the assessment implications of this expansion.

3.2   Assessing Consumer Needs and Preferences

An often overlooked issue in psychology that receives explicit attention in public health is that people with problems and their families and other social network members are *consumers of services*. They make choices to use or not to use help from an array of resources that range from lay helpers, to mutual help groups, to clergy, to life coaches, to nonspecialty health care, to specialty behavioral health services. Some services are provided face-to-face (FTF); others are delivered electronically by email or on the web; and other resources can be found in the self-help section of bookstores. Available resources span the lay and professional sectors, resulting in a "pluralistic" system of care (Wang et al., 2005).

Assessment of consumer needs and preferences can help close the gap between need for, and utilization of, mental health services.

Despite the many options, utilization of MH/SU services continues to lag behind population need (Wang et al., 2005; WHO World Mental Health Survey Consortium, 2004). Remediating this gap depends on identifying and reducing barriers to care, promoting earlier help-seeking before problems become serious, and making behavioral health services more attractive to the consumer base. Without population-specific preference data, however, providers may make erroneous assumptions about attributes of psychological services that appeal to consumers. For instance, a *Consumer Reports* survey concerning MH/SU services (Seligman, 1995) found that consumers preferred lay services like Alcoholics Anonymous over professional treatment. Another survey of preferences for professional, lay, and anonymous computerized and self-help resources for SUDs found that personal help was preferred over more anonymous forms of help, even for these stigmatized disorders (Tucker et al., 2009). However, respondents were indifferent to whether the personalized help was dispensed by professional or lay providers.

Clients, their families, and social network members are consumers of services, with preferences that affect treatment entry, retention, and outcomes.

Such findings draw attention to the need to assess consumer preferences in the design and delivery of behavioral health services. As illustrated above, this can be done by conducting consumer surveys and needs assessments among interested stakeholders. This may include the organizations that fund or deliver services and the social networks and family members of persons with problems, in addition to the end-point consumers of services.

A common, less formal approach is to conduct *focus groups*. Members of the target group or at-risk community are invited to participate in small- to moderate-sized discussion groups typically led by a public health professional to obtain information about consumer needs and preferences (Krueger & Casey, 2008). Preestablished questions are asked in an interactive discussion format. Responses are typically recorded for later review, with nonidentifying respondent characteristics (e.g., race, gender) attached to the comments.

Opinion leaders in the community can be trained to serve as "community health advisors," providing health-related information to their neighbors.

Another way to obtain such information is to interview key opinion leaders in a target community or group. In addition to guiding program development, opinion leaders can be enlisted to help with program dissemination and adoption. *Community health advisors* (CHAs; also referred to as *promotores* or lay health advisors), who typically are respected members of the target population, can be trained in health-related areas of local concern and then asked to provide this information to people in their communities. CHA approaches have had considerable success across health-related issues, including diabetes management, HIV risk reduction, and cardiovascular risk reduction. For example,

CHAs trained in diabetes prevention and reduction strategies provided health information to local churches in African-American communities (Plescia, Herrick, & Chavis, 2008). At follow-up, communities that received the CHA intervention showed significant improvements in fruit and vegetable consumption and physical activity compared with comparable control communities.

Venue enumeration sampling (VES; Muhib et al., 2001) is another systemic technique for identifying channels and venues for community-based interventions. In VES, a list of community-suggested venues is first compiled. Then the number of potential intervention recipients, as well as observable demographic characteristics, such as age and gender, are counted during preselected days and blocks of time at the venues. These data are then used to select locations and sampling frames likely to yield high numbers of potential recipients. A second step is to conduct brief, nonidentifying screening interviews with individuals at these likely high-yield locations and times to verify the number with the characteristics of interest. These data inform final selection of venues, days, and times most likely to yield a significant proportion of individuals with the target characteristics.

Venue enumeration sampling identifies locations, days, and times most likely to allow broad reach into a target population.

Obtaining information on consumer preferences and needs is essential to *social marketing* techniques used in the development and delivery of public health programs to targeted at-risk groups and communities. Social marketing emphasizes client or consumer definitions of problems and solutions, and incorporates this information into program planning and evaluation (Weinreich, 1999). A mix of qualitative and quantitative methods is generally employed. As an example, see the US Centers for Disease Control and Prevention (CDC) VERB campaign to increase physical activity among "tweens" ages 9-13 (Wong et al., 2004). For this campaign, planning and development steps were informed by qualitative interviews, focus groups, secondary research, and phone surveys with tweens, parents, and other adults who were working with youths.

Social marketing is client centered and incorporates client-defined problems and solutions into program planning and evaluation.

The scope of consumer assessment should be multileveled and cover service features that matter to them, such as provider characteristics, cost, and convenience. The organization and financing of health systems can pose barriers to care that can be improved to enhance treatment entry and engagement. For example, substance misusers and their families value convenient appointments, parking, childcare, and onsite HIV-testing as part of substance-related services (Tucker et al., 2009). In addition, time costs related to appointment delays, travel, and waiting in the office deter care-seeking for medical and behavioral health problems (Tucker & Davison, 2000). Treatment entry and retention can be improved by rapid appointments (e.g., same or next day). Remediation of time costs is consistent with IOM (2006) recommendations to improve health care quality.

Organizational and financial barriers, such as long waiting times or limited ability to pay for care, can be addressed through integrated behavioral health programs.

Enterprising clinicians can expand their practices by using these assessment techniques to identify opportunities to reach potential consumers with appealing services, whether they are in care or not, and by improving service delivery features. This consumer-centric approach is common in public health practice and is receiving attention in clinical care. Mental health practitioners who orient their practices in ways that respond to these nonpsychological dimensions of care will be aspiring to meet the six aims of high quality care as defined by the IOM (2001, 2006), which involve safe, effective, patient-centered care that is timely, efficient, and equitable.

3.3   Effective Screening

An optimal continuum of care that ranges from clinical treatment to less inten-sive services such as brief interventions depends on screening to guide rational choices among the array of service options. Effective screening is brief, can be implemented widely across the continuum of risk, and supports case-finding and rapid decision-making about triaging people to brief interventions, spe-cialty care, or further evaluation. Because screening historically has been of limited relevance to clinical practice, many clinicians are unfamiliar with basic screening principles, which we summarize next.

Decisions about whether to screen need to be guided by several consider-ations, and screening should not be conducted under certain conditions. First, if there is no viable preventive, clinical, or palliative intervention available for a particular condition, screening makes little sense from a health, economic, or psychological standpoint, and positive case-findings may have negative ef-fects. For example, genetic screening tests that may reveal future lethal health conditions for which there is no viable treatment (e.g., Huntington's chorea) could create emotional hardship and prejudice insurability, among other con-cerns, and may be contraindicated in some situations.

Second, the design and implementation of screening programs should be informed by the epidemiology of health and behavioral health disorders over individuals' lifespans and by patterns of health care utilization. Effective pro-grams target risk groups and are implemented in venues in which positive cases are likely to be detected in reasonably large numbers. Universal screening programs for whole populations are rare, expensive, and not highly effective, and they may create concerns about privacy, labeling, and false positives when applied to groups or persons with few or no known risk factors. Random drug-testing of entire student bodies in public schools without cause exemplifies these concerns. Although US courts have generally disallowed universal drug-testing, students who represent the public schools (e.g., athletes, participants in extracurricular activities) can be tested "randomly" without specific cause.

Third, screening should be implemented when there is a reasonable likeli-hood that sufficient at-risk or positive cases will be detected to justify the costs of screening and to yield health benefits through early detection and referral to treatment. This is not an easy set of considerations to balance, as illustrated by recent debate over the frequency of mammography for women under age 50. The debate centers on the relative costs of breast cancer screening and treat-ment versus the relatively small numbers of lives saved by annual mammog-raphy prior to age 50. Screening advocates focus on the women whose lives will be saved by mammography, even if the costs of screening and treatment are high. Opponents argue that widespread annual screening is very costly in relation to the low rates of cancer detection in the 40-50 age range for women without breast cancer risk factors (US Preventive Services Task Force, 2009).

Fourth, screening works best when psychometrically sound screening instruments are used that are both sensitive and specific to a given health or behavioral health problem. *Sensitivity* is the extent to which a test identifies true positive cases when disease is present, whereas *specificity* is the extent to which a test avoids yielding false positives when disease is absent (Friis & Sellers, 2003). The best tests have high detection rates of true positives and

Screening supports rapid triage of clients to brief interventions, specialty care, or further evaluation as needed.

Screening is not appropriate if no intervention is available for a given condition.

Programs that target risk groups and locations where priority populations congregate are preferred to universal population screening.

The proportion of at-risk or positive cases likely to be identified should be considered before embarking upon a screening program.

true negatives and very low rates of false positives and misses. In practice, however, most screening tests perform below this ideal. Screening tests need to be brief and often may not have optimal psychometric properties.

A decision to use a given test should be based on its sensitivity and specificity, the various consequences of accurate and inaccurate detection, and the population base rates of the target disorder. Some problems are sufficiently widespread, serious, and treatable that use of an imperfect test is justified. For example, alcohol-related problems are common in medical patients and are important to detect for proper medical management. The four-item CAGE test (an acronym for *cut* down on drinking, *annoyed* by criticism of drinking, *guilty* about drinking, and *eye-opener*) has good sensitivity for identifying medical patients with current alcohol dependence and works well in medical settings where time is short, but it has poor sensitivity for hazardous drinking that does not reach the level of abuse or dependence (Tucker, Murphy, & Kertesz, 2010a).

In other situations, a test that yields a high false positive rate may create new problems, such as mislabeling or avoidance of future screening or treatment, that do not justify its use. For example, premenopausal women under age 50 tend to have dense breast tissue that yields a higher false positive rate than in older women, and repeated false alarms may deter future use of mammography at older ages when breast cancer risk is higher and detection is more accurate (US Preventive Services Task Force, 2009).

Finally, screening procedures need to be easy for nonspecialists and busy professionals to use as a basis of rapid decision-making. Some positive cases will need to be referred to other agencies and professionals for further assessment and treatment. In other cases, the person conducting the screening will provide a brief intervention (e.g., primary care and emergency department providers). Although well-crafted SBI programs can yield health benefits and reduce health care costs (US Preventive Services Task Force, 2004), provider adoption and diffusion of SBIs into general practice remain incomplete. For example, despite the availability of good SBIs for alcohol disorders, they are used by only a minority of US physicians in nonspecialty settings (Tucker et al., 2010a). Table 5 provides a list of websites that present sound screening instruments and procedures for common MH/SU problems.

The ideal screening instrument has high detection rates for true positives and low false positive labeling of persons who are free from disease.

A test with a high false positive rate may create new problems such as mislabeling or future avoidance of screening.

Screening should be brief and simple for providers who have limited time and specialty knowledge.

Table 5
Websites with Screening Tools for Prevalent Behavioral Health Problems

Substance use disorders
- http://www.projectcork.org/clinical_tools/
  10 brief screening tools for alcohol and substance use disorders
- http://www.who.int/substance_abuse/activities/sbi/en/index.html
  The WHO AUDIT for brief assessment of alcohol use disorders
- http://pubs.niaaa.nih.gov/publications/practitioner/PocketGuide/pocket_guide.htm
  NIAAA Pocket Guide for Alcohol Screening and Brief Intervention, 2005 edition
- http://www.who.int/substance_abuse/activities/assist/en/index.html
  ASSIST instrument for brief assessment of alcohol, tobacco and other substance use

Table 5
continued

HIV/AIDS
- http://kap.samhsa.gov/products/brochures/pdfs/tip37_pocket_tool.pdf
  SAMSHA Pocket Tool for clinicians to use in harm reduction and prevention discussions
- http://www.turningpoint.org.au/library/bbv_traq_sv_0606.pdf
  The Blood Borne Virus Transmission Risk Assessment Questionnaire – Short Version

Time horizons
- http://www.thetimeparadox.com/surveys/
  The Zimbardo Time Perspective Inventory and Transcendental-Future Time Perspective Inventory

Depression
- http://depression-primarycare.org/clinicians/toolkits/
  Nine-Item Depression Scale of the Personal Health Questionnaire (PHQ-9)
- http://www.caps.ucsf.edu/tools/surveys/pdf/CopingSelf-EfficacyScale.pdf
  Coping Self-Efficacy Scale

Anxiety
- http://www.fpnotebook.com/Psych/Exam/HmltnAnxtyScl.htm
  This site for primary care providers includes the Hamilton Anxiety Scale (1959)

Nutrition and exercise
- http://www.uri.edu/research/cprc/measures.htm#Weight%20Control
  Scales for transtheoretical model constructs related to weight control, exercise, and a variety of other behaviors, from the Cancer Prevention Research Center
- http://www.des.emory.edu/mfp/ExerciseSEChinese.pdf
  Bandura's Exercise Self-efficacy Scale (ESES)

Note. NIAAA = National Institute on Alcohol Abuse and Alcoholism; ASSIST = Alcohol, Smoking and Substance Involvement Screening Test.

3.4   Assessing Motivation and Readiness to Change

Motivation to change
is not necessarily the
same as motivation
to seek treatment.

Integrated
behavioral health
programs can be
used to support self-
change.

Public health and clinical practitioners are both interested in people's motivation and readiness for change, but they diverge in how they conceptualize and assess it. For example, many clinicians continue to be influenced by early psychoanalytic concepts about motivation, wherein motivation for change was considered synonymous with motivation to seek treatment, and intrinsic motivation was considered superior to extrinsic motivation for psychotherapy. Research findings have substantially modified this view, although it still persists. First, the presence of many external and few internal sources of motivation in the context of help-seeking does not mean that recipients will not benefit from interventions (Tucker & Davison, 2000). Second, natural "self-change" outside the context of treatment is a common occurrence for many behavior problems (Klingemann & Sobell, 2007). This has led to necessary distinctions between motivation to seek services and motivation to change problem behaviors, which are not always the same; e.g., stigmatizing and other negative consequences of seeking treatment can deter or delay treatment entry even when motivation for change is high.

In contrast to clinical concern with individual motivation and treatment-produced change, public health strategies are concerned with reaching at-risk market segments at times when they are receptive to health-oriented messages and interventions, or with using such programs to promote receptivity and readiness to change. As discussed next, this opportunistic, active approach is quite different from the passive clinical approach of waiting for motivated clients to find their way into a clinician's office.

3.4.1   Finding and Using Teachable Moments

Finding the right time, venue, and method to screen and intervene requires consideration of practical, empirical, and conceptual issues. A classic public health example is requiring up-to-date vaccinations for children as they enter day care or public school. The timing of the requirement is responsive to the need to protect schools as a whole from the spread of communicable diseases. This policy also employs a practical time and channel to reach deep into the population of children when parents are required by law to educate their off-spring.

Population approaches actively seek out "teachable moments" and opportunities to plant the idea and tools of behavior change.

Behavioral health practitioners need to consider these same kinds of issues and opportunities in light of the evidence on behavior change, screening and intervention costs, venue and time selection to reach large numbers of persons, and effective health communication strategies. This requires a sound working knowledge of the population dynamics of behavioral health problems, including when and where persons with different risk factors or problems will surface and be receptive to behavioral health screenings and services. A good example of how to address these issues effectively is screening emergency department patients who have accidental injuries (e.g., vehicular or boating accidents, falls) for alcohol misuse, which is common in such injuries, and then providing brief interventions or treatment referrals as indicated (NIAAA, 2005; Tucker et al., 2010a).

Good health communication practices are especially important because, without them, an otherwise well designed, timed, and implemented behavioral health intervention that reaches its market segment will not be heard and adopted by the target audience. For example, cancer patients in hospital settings may benefit from health education and behavioral interventions aimed at managing pain and maintaining mobility, nutrition, and other positive health behaviors during and after treatment. Although the target audience is large and accessible, the timing of behavioral health programs is challenging because cancer patients frequently are acutely ill, anxious, or in pain, and their ability to uptake otherwise beneficial information and services can be compromised at such times. Some familiarity with the research on health communications, as well as the kinds of variables that influence whether recipients use the information they receive, is essential for identifying and using good teachable moments in ways that promote positive health behaviors and outcomes. As

---

Biases in Health Decision-Making

Behavioral economic studies have shown that health and affective states influence health decision-making in complex ways that can guide the timing of opportunistic behavioral health programs (Tucker et al., 2010b). When people are in "hot" emotional or deprived states (e.g., hungry or in pain), they tend to respond more to the present circumstances and discount future health outcomes to a greater degree than when they are in "cold" states (Loewenstein, 2005a). In hot states, they also tend to overestimate the stability of their current preferences over time, whereas in cold states, they fail to appreciate how much their hot states influence their preferences and behavior. This pattern is important because medical decisions are often made when people are in a hot state after receiving bad health news or when they are in pain or discomfort.

Higher discounting of future health-related outcomes is also associated with poor health status, and individuals also tend to project their current preferences onto future choices when they should be irrelevant (Loewenstein, 2005b). This *projection bias* causes people to exaggerate the duration of current unpleasant feelings and to take actions with long-term consequences based on their short-term preferences. See Tucker et al. (2010b) for discussion of other sources of bias in health decision-making.

---

one example, the text box discusses how health and affective states can influence health communication and medical decision-making, using findings from behavioral economic studies.

3.4.2   Stage of Change

Several questionnaires guided by the TTM are available to assess the stage of change of individuals with different psychological and behavioral health problems (Tucker et al., 2010a). Some scales are generic, and others are disorder-specific. An example of a generic scale that asks about problems in a general way is the original University of Rhode Island Change Assessment (URICA; McConnaughy, Prochaska, & Velicer, 1983) . The single item Readiness Ruler, developed for use in motivational interviewing programs (Rollnick, Miller, & Butler, 2008), provides a current assessment of how ready clients are to change problem behaviors. Clients rate how ready they are to change on a 10-point scale, where 1 = *definitely not ready to change* and 10 = *definitely ready to change*. This simple rating guides subsequent discussion of change goals and possibilities, and it can be repeated to assess changes in motivation. The similar Contemplation Ladder (Biener & Abrams, 1991), developed for use in smoking cessation programs, also involves a single rating of motivation to change (0 = "*no thought of changing my [problem behavior]*" to 10 = "*taking action to change*"). Both provide a continuous measure that can be used to track motivation to change.

> **Questionnaires are available to stage individuals by readiness to change behaviors. The findings can be used to tailor interventions.**

Such scales assess where individuals are in the change process, for purposes of delivering an intervention that is matched to the stage of change. Despite the appeal of this matching approach, research is mixed regarding the utility of such scales to predict outcomes of behavior change attempts. For example, it is not clear that people in a change process move through the discrete stages in a sequential manner as posited by the TTM, and stage assignments across measures have been somewhat discordant (Napper et al., 2008).

3.4.3   Temporal Dynamics of Motivation and Change

Measures of individuals' temporal sensitivity to delayed outcomes have been found to discriminate between persons who do and do not engage in high-risk health behaviors, such as alcohol and drug misuse, risky sex, and failure to use seat belts (Bickel & Marsch, 2000; Zimbardo & Boyd, 2008). Such "time horizon" measures also predict outcomes of treatment and natural recovery attempts for several behavioral health problems (Tucker et al., 2010b). Thus, characterizing the extent to which individuals orient their behavior around present versus future goals is relevant to developing change goals and strategies that work with clients' patterns of behavioral organization. For many problems, the goal is to support short-term change for a sufficient interval for clients to make contact with delayed valued activities and outcomes that will maintain positive behavior change longer-term.

Questionnaires such as the Zimbardo Time Perspective Inventory (ZTPI; Zimbardo & Boyd, 2008) and the Consideration of Future Consequences scale (CFC; Strathman, Gleicher, Boninger, & Edwards, 1994) assess the extent to which people orient their lives toward the past, present, or future. Substance misusers and those engaged in other risky behaviors tend to have more present-oriented and less future-oriented perspectives compared with normal controls (Zimbardo & Boyd, 2008). Computerized and questionnaire "delay discounting" tasks have shown similar relationships between temporal preferences and substance use patterns (Bickel & Marsch, 2000; Tucker et al., 2010b). Appendix 1 includes the brief 12-item CFC questionnaire. See Zimbardo and Boyd, 2008, for the ZPTI and scoring instructions, and see http://www.thetimeparadox.com/surveys/ for an online version.

> **Individuals engaged in risky behaviors often are more present-oriented and less future-oriented in their time horizons.**

3.4.4   Self-Efficacy and Contextual Factors

Extratherapeutic contextual factors influence the change process from initiation through maintenance and relapse. Self-efficacy expectations are well-established predictors of behavioral outcomes that are context-specific, and scales for different behavior problems assess the extent to which individuals believe they can perform behaviors essential to the change process in specific high-risk situations (Tucker et al., 2010a). For example, self-efficacy to reduce substance use can be assessed using the 10-item version of the Situational Confidence Questionnaire (Breslin, Sobell, Sobell, & Agrawal, 2000), and HIV-related self-efficacy and outcome expectations can be assessed using a scale designed by Semple, Patterson, and Grant (2000). Higher baseline self-efficacy predicts better behavioral outcomes; treatment can modify self-efficacy; and higher posttreatment self-efficacy is correlated with good outcomes.

> **Self-efficacy is a strong predictor of context-specific outcomes, and scales are available for a variety of behaviors.**

3.5   Moving From Screening and Assessment to Intervention

Effective integration of clinical and public health practices rests on using knowledge about the behavioral epidemiology of MH/SU disorders and about patterns and influences on care-seeking to design and implement screening and intervention programs for targeted risk groups. This population perspective builds on knowledge of clinical diagnostic systems, such as those of the *Diagnostic and Statistical Manual of Mental Disorders* (DSM) and *International Classification of Diseases* (ICD), in concert with knowledge of the distribution of MH/SU disorders. Prevalence of a given disorder ranges from subclinical to clinically diagnosable variations in different health care and community settings and varies across demographic and socioeconomic groups. These base rates should guide target selection and program development.

> **Effective assessment lays the foundation for effective intervention.**

Effective behavioral health practitioners will need to be familiar with barriers to seeking care in the specialty and general health care sectors. This requires that clinicians supplement their training and continuing education with materials such as those presented in this book that place their clinical activities within a population-based public health context grounded in the behavioral epidemiology of MH/SU disorders and the associated patterns of help-seeking and service utilization. Behavioral health practitioners will need a working knowledge of the venues and circumstances in which people with different problems of varying severity are likely to surface and to be receptive to suitable interventions. Finding opportunities for early case-finding and intervention delivery in health care systems, worksites, schools, churches, and other community settings is a basic tactic of public health practice and extends the reach and potential impact of behavioral health care. Rapid assessment of individuals' behavioral health problems, and triaging them accordingly, are key components of service delivery to a broader range of clients than those who seek specialty MH/SU care. Comprehensive implementation of a population perspective requires assessment of the motivations and life circumstances of potential recipients of care at the time contact is made with them.

> **Knowledge of the broader context will help overcome barriers to treatment and allow targeted implementation of interventions.**

Select services built on this intervention strategy are discussed in Chapter 4. They range from low-technology interventions using print materials to telephone- and computer-based interventions that employ contemporary communications systems to deliver behavioral health messages that can be individualized with varying specificity. We focus on these services suggested by strategies and tactics of public health practice because they can bridge the clinic–community interface and are within reach of many mental health practitioners. They share some common concepts and procedures with familiar FTF interventions that "meet clients where they are," such as motivational interviewing (Miller & Rollnick, 2002), but they can be disseminated more easily to larger numbers of persons.

4

Treatment

4.1 Using Media and Technology to Extend the Scope of Practice

Historically, face-to-face (FTF) psychotherapy has been the most widely used, efficacious treatment in the mental health professions. One challenge associated with FTF services is the prohibitive cost of widespread translation and dissemination. FTF interventions require substantial personnel time, training, and financial support for sustainability. Public health interventions may be less expensive to develop, implement, and sustain, but historically they have lacked the capacity to individualize intervention messages. Recent advances in computer and communications technologies offer clinicians and researchers unprecedented opportunity to create and deliver client-centered interventions that may improve the public's health and overall quality of life (Graham & Abrams, 2005). This chapter describes these services, which vary in their reach into the population in need and in their degree of individualization. Services discussed include print materials; interactive voice response (IVR) and cell phone applications; and high-technology internet, other personal computer, and expert system interventions.

> **Advances in technology have significantly increased our ability to customize population interventions and increase reach and impact.**

None of these services involve much, if any, FTF contact with a mental health professional, although many can be used to supplement FTF services. The interventions also vary in the extent to which they use information about individuals or groups to create an intervention to match their specific characteristics or needs: (1) *Generic* interventions provide general information and action-oriented behavior change messages and have often been considered a standard public health intervention; (2) *Personalized* interventions use specific characteristics of a person such as his or her name and add it to generic material so as to appear more personal; (3) *Targeted* interventions are developed with a certain segment of the population in mind, such as women, adolescents, or the elderly, and the content reflects certain aspects of the target subgroup; and (4) *Tailored* interventions are individualized for a specific person and are fairly analogous to a FTF intervention, even if the delivery channel is not in-person (Noar, Benac, & Harris, 2007). In other words, tailored interventions are designed to simulate personal counseling (IOM, 2003).

> **Targeted interventions are customized to a subpopulation. Tailored interventions are customized to the individual.**

Effective tailoring is central to many of these new practice tools for behavioral health care. In a typical application, an individual is assessed by questionnaire, and the responses are used to generate individualized feedback and therapeutic instruction related to the outcome of interest, ideally grounded in

Tailoring typically involves using a person's assessment responses to generate individualized feedback and therapeutic instruction.

established behavior change theory (IOM 2003; Noar, Black, & Pierce, 2009). Tailored information is more appealing, tends to be read more deeply, and is viewed as personally relevant by end users. As a result, they are more likely to act upon the information.

Advances in behavioral science and technology have allowed for true customization of health messages, and a variety of potentially cost-effective delivery channels that are described in this chapter can be used as "stand alone" interventions or as adjuncts to FTF interventions. These intervention modalities and delivery channels can be used to provide the public with personal behavioral health services and access to preventive care that otherwise would be unavailable. Such practices exemplify a core ethical principle of public health that basic health resources should be available to all. Appendices 2 and 3 provide lists of self-guided change and behavioral intervention websites, respectively.

4.2 Methods of Treatment

4.2.1 Print Interventions

Description

Print interventions are simple, inexpensive, accessible, and moderately efficacious. However, literacy can be a concern.

Print materials such as pamphlets, newsletters, magazines, letters, manuals, and booklets regarding specific behaviors or conditions have been widely used in public health programs and have generally been considered "low-intensity" interventions. Although their content is often generic, print materials also can be personalized, targeted, or tailored (Kreuter, Strecher, & Glassman, 1999). Bibliotherapy is another form of print intervention that can be used as a self-directed stand-alone intervention or as an adjunct to FTF interventions. Table 6 summarizes the strengths and weaknesses of print applications.

Use simple language, terms, and visual aids in print interventions that recipients can understand and do not find offensive or culturally inappropriate.

In all applications, it is vital to use simple language, terms, and visual aids that recipients can understand and do not find offensive or culturally inappropriate. Many effective mail brochures can be found online. For example, mental health brochures can be found at http://www.RightHealth.com; immunization brochures in 24 different languages can be found at http://ethnomed.org/patient-education/immunization/immunization. Also see the CDC website for the *Five a Day* nutrition program (http://www.fruitsandveggiesmatter.

Table 6
Print Materials for Behavioral Health Interventions

- Low technology
- Typically generic, but can be personalized or tailored
- Universal, selective, and indicated prevention
- Adjunct to professional care
- Typically mailed; can be hand delivered or distributed at high-traffic locations (e.g., waiting rooms)
- Relatively inexpensive with good reach into the population
- Dependent on recipient literacy; receipt and use often hard to verify

gov/) and the US National Institute of Drug Abuse (NIDA) drug prevention website for students and young adults (http://www.drugabuse.gov/students.html).

Mechanisms of Action

Print materials tend to have fairly small effect sizes (Cohen's $d = 0.07$ to 0.34) contingent upon the target behavior, use of pictures and graphics, and/or the type of print material employed (generic, personal, targeted, or tailored). (*Note:* Effect sizes are defined as the standardized mean difference between a treatment and control condition on an outcome variable; $d \leq 0.3$, 0.5, or 0.7 are indicative of small, medium, and large effect sizes.) Despite their small effect sizes, print materials are relatively inexpensive to implement, and their reach into the population is potentially very broad. If received by recipients in need at a teachable moment, they promote behavior change at the individual level that, when summed over the population, can have a measurable impact on aggregate health status.

For example, in a randomized controlled trial (RCT) concerned with reaching untreated problem drinkers in US communities to promote self-change from drinking problems (Sobell et al., 2002), a generic print brochure resulted in positive changes in drinking from baseline levels over a 1-year follow-up that were similar to a more personalized guided self-change intervention that included drinking feedback and motivational materials based on individual assessment. Interestingly, many of the 800 problem drinker participants stopped misusing alcohol around the time they saw the study recruitment advertisement stating that natural recovery was possible and decided to call to participate. Finding such teachable moments and timing the delivery of relevant health messages accordingly is basic to the effectiveness of such opportunistic interventions to facilitate change.

> Timing delivery of lower intensity interventions to take advantage of "teachable moments" can elicit behavior change without costly treatment.

Efficacy and Prognosis

A meta-analysis of self-help for anxiety and depression (den Boer, Wiersma, & Van Den Bosch, 2004) that included 13 studies involving bibliotherapy, based primarily on cognitive behavior therapy (CBT), found a mean effect size of $d = 0.84$ posttreatment for self-help versus waiting list or attention placebo control conditions ($d = 0.76$ at follow-up). The mean effect size of self-help versus FTF CBT was -0.03 posttreatment (-0.07 at follow-up). Bibliotherapy thus performed significantly better than no treatment and only marginally worse than FTF treatment.

Although most print interventions are considered minimal interventions, those providing tailored information and messages based on specific variables related to an individual are more effective. In a meta-analysis of 57 studies that compared tailored and untailored print materials in studies that variously focused on smoking cessation, dietary change, and mammography screening (Noar et al., 2007), some degree of tailoring generally improved outcomes over untailored print materials. The results showed a small sample size–weighted mean effect size ($r = 0.074$; 95% confidence interval [CI] = 0.066, 0.082) for the tailored print interventions, which significantly outperformed the nontailored materials. (*Note*: Pearson's r can be used to report effect sizes for nonexperimental data.)

> Tailored print materials are more efficacious than generic materials. Pamphlets, newsletters, and magazines are preferred over letters, manuals, or booklets.

The most successful print materials were pamphlets, newsletters, and magazines, as opposed to letters, manuals, or booklets. However, because few publications provided details about the "look" or layout of materials, Noar et al. (2007) speculated that the use of pictures and graphics along with text in the pamphlets, newsletters, and magazines may have resulted in better retention and use of the information, and therefore better outcomes.

Variations and Combinations of Methods

The distribution of print materials can vary by channel, frequency, venue, and target audience. Print materials can be mailed, emailed, or handed out to recipients (e.g., in shopping malls, at sporting events, or at community festivals) and can be made available at hospitals, pharmacies, or other health services agencies, often in patient waiting areas. Using multiple dissemination channels is optimal in some applications. Print materials can be distributed all at once, or distributed several times over longer periods, e.g., on a rotating basis to different segments of a target community until coverage is "saturated."

Consider theory, target behavior, audience, tailoring requirements, and cost when deciding how to distribute print materials.

Decisions about how to distribute print materials should be guided by behavior change theory, the target behavior, audience characteristics, level of tailoring, and cost. As discussed in Chapter 3, low-threshold, opportunistic interventions such as print materials are more likely to promote positive change when they reach at-risk recipients at a teachable moment when they are receptive to behavioral health information and the possibility of change. Information alone is rarely sufficient to promote behavior change in the absence of motivation to change and the resources to do it. The optimal combination of channel, frequency, venue, target audience, and receptivity will vary across behavioral health problems and should be informed by epidemiological data about patterns of risk and health-seeking in the target audience.

Identification of high-yield venues and channels is crucial to success of print and other low intensity interventions.

Another basic step in effective print interventions is identifying the venues and channels that yield the highest percentage of at-risk recipients. This can be relatively straightforward in some organizational settings, e.g., distributing breast cancer screening information to female patients in obstetrics-gynecology clinics. For some community-based interventions, appropriate channels and venues can be identified through the use of focus groups, interviews with lay and professional health opinion leaders, or venue enumeration sampling, as described in Chapter 3. Regardless of the method used, obtaining data at the locations, days, and times most likely to yield high numbers of individuals with the target characteristics is fundamental to sound intervention planning and delivery.

Problems With Carrying Out Print Interventions

Print materials should be written at a fifth to seventh grade level to ensure comprehension by the widest audience possible.

Print materials obviously cannot be used by persons who cannot read due to literacy, visual, or cognitive impairments. Many print materials are too complex for nearly half of US adults to understand and use (IOM, 2003). The general rule of thumb is that all text should be written at the fifth to seventh grade reading level. The inclusion of graphics, pictures, and symbols to reinforce text is helpful and, like text, can also be personalized or tailored. When developing the layout and overall look, as well as selecting colors, the cultural preferences of the target population should be kept in mind.

Another concern is that there is no easy way to verify that intended recipients received, much less read or used, print materials. Mass mailings are a scattershot approach to universal prevention, and some selection of recipients (e.g., by postal code, employer, school district, or church membership) is helpful, although obtaining more specific information upon which to select recipients can raise privacy concerns. Whether the health-related print materials come by mail or email, they need to be designed in such a way that recipients do not consider them to be junk mail or spam.

Multicultural Issues

Print interventions can be prepared in any written language using visual aids that have meaning for different ethnic, racial, gender, and age groups, among other individual differences that may be relevant to effective health communication. Even generic print materials should be prepared with the intended population in mind, using basic principles of sound health communication: Use pictures of actors who look like the intended audience, use health-promoting rather than fear-based motivational messages, and make clear action statements (NCI, 2001). An experienced health educator familiar with the intended audience should review the print materials for reading level, appropriate terminology, and the like. A graphic artist can be helpful because the use of pictures and graphics along with text appears to increase retention and use of written health-related information (Noar et al., 2007).

> Use health-promoting messages rather than fear-based appeals to encourage change.

4.2.2   Interactive Voice Response (IVR) Systems

Description

Table 7 summarizes the main features of IVR and other cellular phone applications. IVR systems are an automated form of telephone communication that has widespread behavioral health utility because the vast majority of most populations have phone access. This includes persons who live in disadvantaged rural or inner-city areas that are underserved by medical and MH/SU services and who lack personal computer access or literacy. For this reason, IVR systems deserve wider usage in systems of care that seek to reach from the clinic into the community and expand therapeutic and prevention programs (Abu-Hasaballah et al., 2007).

> Even if a population has low literacy, limited computer access, and few professional providers, most members will have telephone access.

IVR systems connect telephone users to a computerized data collection and storage system that asks callers to respond to prerecorded questions with response options that callers typically enter using a touch-tone phone keypad. Caller responses are entered directly into electronic data files that can be checked automatically, thereby eliminating data entry time and costs and greatly reducing input errors. Because no verbal reports are required in touch-tone IVR systems, caller responses are private, which is conducive to reporting sensitive information (Abu-Hasaballah et al., 2007; Schroder & Johnson, 2009). This aspect of IVR systems has made them appealing in applications that involve sensitive and stigmatized behaviors, such as addictive behaviors, risky sexual practices, and mental disorders. Speech recognition software is also available to transcribe callers' audioresponses but is not optimal for most behavioral health applications due to the risk of responses being overheard.

Table 7
Telephone-Based Approaches for Behavioral Health Interventions

Interactive voice response (IVR) applications
- Low technology for end users; medium to high for providers
- Supports tailoring and individual feedback, ongoing assessment
- Selective and indicated prevention
- Stand-alone or adjunct to professional care
- End users access system by phone; providers set up and maintain IVR hardware, software and phone lines, and data files
- Broad reach (near-universal phone access); private; convenient; low cost for users; allows real-time interactions and reports; enhances sensitive reports; minimal user literacy required
- Provider start-up costs high: hardware, software, programming, management; for some projects, outsourcing may reduce provider costs

Cellular phone applications
- Low technology for end users; medium to high for providers
- Supports tailoring and individual feedback, ongoing assessment
- Selective and indicated prevention
- Stand-alone or adjunct to professional care
- End users access system by phone; providers set up and maintain hardware, software and phone lines, and data files
- Broad reach (rapid cell phone adoption); convenient; low cost for users; allows real-time interactions and reports; more flexible than IVR; offers web access, graphics, etc.; minimal user literacy required
- Provider start-up costs high: hardware, software, programming, management; for some projects, outsourcing may reduce provider costs
- Not as private/secure for end user

IVR systems can be used for assessment, monitoring, and intervention either as the sole platform or to supplement in-person care.

With advances in IVR software, system features have become increasingly flexible and useful for behavioral health applications, including assessment, long-term monitoring of chronic health and behavioral health problems, and serving as a platform for intervention delivery (Abu-Hasaballah et al., 2007; Schroder & Johnson, 2009). IVR systems have been used as a stand-alone assessment or intervention approach, as an adjunct to in-person professional care, or phased in as an aftercare service when treatment is ending. Newer IVR software supports programming to make reminder calls about appointments, medication usage, and other time-sensitive behaviors important for health management. IVR systems can be programmed to alert clinic staff (e.g., via pager or email) when a client enters information that requires immediate attention, such as reports of suicidal thoughts or domestic violence.

IVR data collected from individuals over time can be used to provide tailored feedback and behavior change instructions either as part of ongoing IVR calls or as graphs of key behaviors and outcomes that are mailed or emailed to callers (e.g., Helzer et al., 2008). For example, IVR data have been used successfully to provide feedback and support to informal caregivers of community-dwelling persons with Alzheimer's disease (Mahoney, Tarlow, & Jones, 2003). IVR interventions can be personalized and integrated with ongoing monitoring of behaviors, mood states, and outcomes of interest, such as dietary changes (e.g., Glasgow, Christensen, Smith, Stevens, & Toobert, 2009) and chronic pain symptoms (Naylor, Keefe, Brigidi, Naud, & Helzer, 2008).

IVR systems have utility for monitoring and managing chronic health and behavioral health problems, including relapsing-remitting disorders such as SUDs. They can be made available to clients over long periods, serving to promote risk detection and relapse prevention (e.g., Mundt, Moore, & Bean, 2006) and rapid treatment reentry as needed. IVR systems thus are a prototypic "extensive" intervention that can extend care beyond the limited duration of a course of "intensive" psychotherapy (Humphreys & Tucker, 2002). The text box illustrates an extensive IVR application from our work with untreated problem drinkers that makes IVR self-monitoring (SM) available as they seek to resolve drinking problems on their own.

IVR software has become less costly and easier to program for use with inexpensive personal computers (PCs) equipped with telephone interface cards that route calls to electronic data collection and storage files (e.g., SmartQ/ DialQ; Telesage Inc., Chapel Hill, NC, USA). PC-based IVR systems are powerful and flexible enough for most research and practice applications. Large-group applications with heavy system access and data storage needs (e.g., as part of a state-level MCO) may find outsourcing to commercial IVR businesses preferable (Abu-Hasaballah et al., 2007).

Using IVR Self-Monitoring to Support Natural Resolution of Drinking Problems in Community-Dwelling Adults

---

Most problem drinkers do not seek professional treatment. Many initiate quit attempts on their own, and the risk of relapse is high during the first 3–6 months when new sober behavior patterns are emerging and are not yet stable. This is an opportunity to use an interactive voice response (IVR) platform to provide an "extensive" intervention to support natural resolution outside of the health system.

As part of an ongoing randomized controlled trial (RCT) comparing IVR-assisted and unaided natural resolution attempts, recently resolved community-dwelling problem drinkers in the United States received daily access to IVR self-monitoring (SM) for 6 months. After initial face-to-face (FTF) training, they called a toll-free number and engaged in daily SM of urges to drink, alcohol use, and other behavioral and contextual factors involved in stabilizing or destabilizing resolutions. Appendix 4 shows a subset of the daily IVR questions about drinking. Additional intervention elements were build around the IVR protocol, including weekly IVR-delivered brief education modules that followed a typical course of recovery; e.g., early topics pertained to drinking goal setting and relapse prevention, and later topics pertained to making changes in other areas of life-health functioning that support stable resolutions (e.g., nondrinking social networks, sound money management). A workbook accompanied the weekly education modules and included homework assignments.

Each month during the IVR SM interval, participants received a personalized feedback letter that summarized their IVR calling patterns, reinforced high IVR utilization, and included graphs summarizing daily drinking prior to resolution and as reported postresolution via IVR SM. Appendix 5 shows graphs for one participant. These materials illustrate how IVR systems can be used to support a lengthy behavior change process embedded in individuals' ongoing life contexts.

Mechanisms of Action

The mechanisms of IVR action likely vary somewhat across the different applications spanning assessment, feedback, interventions, and remote ambulatory monitoring. It is incumbent upon the practitioner to determine whether an evidence-based FTF clinical procedure has also been evaluated positively using the IVR format (Abu-Hasaballah et al., 2007). For example, when established paper or interview assessments are converted to an IVR format, the IVR scripts need to be piloted to assure that they yield proper response data.

IVR systems have unique qualities that likely influence the mechanisms of action in more general ways. First, IVR systems obviously do not have the capacity for therapist empathy that is a basic mechanism of action of effective psychotherapy and motivational interviewing (Miller & Rollnick, 2002). However, this is not as serious a limitation as it may seem. When using the IVR to supplement FTF care, the therapist can record the IVR script and verbal statements to reinforce key reports on the IVR. Also, most IVR applications require an initial FTF session to train callers how to use the system, during which rapport can be established to motivate IVR use over the coming weeks and months. The use of feedback letters and graphs of clients' IVR data can further solidify a "working" relationship between providers and clients, even if mediated through the IVR system (Helzer et al., 2008). In our experience and that of others (e.g., Schroder & Johnson, 2009), clients often come to regard the IVR as a form of communication with the therapist or person who trained them to use the IVR, and some want to continue using the IVR after a protocol ends.

A second feature of IVR systems that can serve as a mechanism of change rests on the utility to support client reports of sensitive information in a private, confidential context. This aspect can be beneficial both for accurate data collection and for aiding clients' problem identification and resolution. Journaling is known to have therapeutic benefits, and the IVR can be used as a form of ongoing personal disclosure and analysis.

Third, SM using IVR or other recording systems can promote reductions in the behaviors being reported. Although often viewed as a nuisance variable by researchers ("measurement reactivity"), the reactive effects of SM are advantageous in behavior change programs. The reductions may not be long-lasting, but they offer an opportunity to promote alternative functional behaviors in the natural environments in which problem behaviors occur. SM also supports self-observation and development of problem-solving skills.

Conceptually, SM is regarded as an integral part of effective behavioral self-regulation and is thought to highlight perceptions of a discrepancy between current *discrete acts* and long-term *patterns of behavior* that vary in value (Rachlin, 1995). Behavior patterns with delayed positive consequences are often more valuable as a whole compared with discrete behaviors chosen day-to-day, even though, on any given day, the discrete behavior (e.g., smoking, risky sex) may be highly preferred. Drawing attention to the delayed consequences of behavior patterns or signaling their future availability via SM (or another discrepancy-inducing interventions such as motivational interviewing), is thought to promote behavior change by helping people frame their day-to-day choices as part of an extended series of linked behaviors, events, and outcomes with higher overall value (Rachlin, 1995).

When converting paper instruments to IVR format, pilot test to assure that proper response data are generated.

Clients sometimes see IVR use as a form of communication with the therapist or IVR trainer.

IVR can afford a greater sense of privacy than FTF interviews for reporting sensitive information.

Self-monitoring with IVR can promote positive behavior change.

IVR self-monitoring can draw attention to both good and bad delayed consequences of health behaviors.

Efficacy and Prognosis

Evidence concerning IVR efficacy and effectiveness comes from four areas: (1) consumer satisfaction studies, (2) findings of reactive effects on target behaviors, (3) evidence for higher reports of sensitive, complex information using IVR systems, and (4) controlled trials that evaluated IVR-based intervention components on outcomes.

Consumer Satisfaction: IVR systems have been well received by end users, including in applications for substance abuse, obsessive-compulsive disorders, diabetes, HIV/AIDS, exercise and medication adherence, among others (Abu-Hasaballah et al., 2007), including in applications with the economically disadvantaged. This is important because consumer satisfaction increases utilization, retention, and outcomes of health and MH/SU services.

Reactive Effects of SM: Although debate continues about the magnitude and persistence of its reactive effects, SM reduces problem behaviors at least for a time, an effect that has been exploited for therapeutic purposes for many disorders (e.g., Miller & Wilbourne, 2002). Early research suggested greater reductions from SM on negative than positive behaviors and that tracking multiple behaviors at once tended to reduce the reactive effects of SM on any given behavior (Hayes & Cavoir, 1980). More recent work has shown that SM remains a valuable component of behavioral interventions, even if evidence for its stand-alone therapeutic efficacy is mixed (e.g., Barta et al., 2008; Helzer et al., 2008). For example, a review of RCTs of alcohol treatments (Miller & Wilbourne, 2002) ranked SM 10th with respect to positive evidence for clinical efficacy among 46 modalities evaluated in 361 clinical trials. Modalities ranked below SM included cognitive therapy, self-control training, and relapse prevention, among more than 30 others.

Enhanced Reporting of Sensitive Information: IVR and similar electronic data collection systems result in higher, presumably more complete reports of sensitive, complex information compared with structured interviews or self-administered questionnaires (Abu-Hasaballah et al., 2007; Schroder & Johnson, 2009). The apparently higher quality of IVR reports is likely due to the privacy it affords and the near real-time data collection it supports. This beneficial feature may be advantageous for reaching underserved population subgroups that avoid or delay clinical care because their problems are sensitive and stigmatized (e.g., rural or economically disadvantaged persons living with HIV/AIDS).

Controlled Intervention Trials: Positive outcomes of IVR SM have been shown for weight management (e.g., Glasgow et al., 2009), chronic pain management after FTF CBT (e.g., Naylor et al., 2008), and mental health problems such as obsessive-compulsive disorder (e.g., Greist et al., 2002). Findings for IVR applications for HIV risk reduction and alcohol problems are mixed. For example, sexually active college students who engaged in IVR SM over 3 months reported reductions in risky sex over time, whereas other trials found no significant decreases (Schroder & Johnson, 2009). Mundt et al. (2006) implemented IVR SM as an aftercare relapse prevention strategy following residential alcohol treatment and found that IVR participants reported better drinking outcomes at 6 months compared with a control group without IVR access. However, frequent reminders calls when participants did not use the IVR system did not promote use and were associated with higher dropout

> **IVR systems have been well received by users in a wide variety of behavioral health applications.**

> **Outcomes for many conditions improve with IVR-based interventions, but results for HIV risk and alcohol problems are mixed.**

rates. Helzer et al. (2008) evaluated IVR SM with primary care patients with alcohol problems and did not find clear evidence for improved outcomes as a function of IVR access.

Prognosis: Similar to other lower intensity interventions (e.g., motivational interviewing), IVR SM appears sufficient to promote stable positive change among persons with mild to moderate behavioral health problems. IVR SM also has utility for persons with more serious problems who need long-term monitoring and linkages to care, but it is not recommended as a stand-alone intervention when FTF clinical treatment is needed. Rather, the utility of IVR applications lies in reaching beyond the clinic into the community to connect with underserved population segments that avoid or delay clinical care, or in its use with patient groups that have chronic disorders. For example, caring for patients with Alzheimer's disease in the home rather than in long-term care facilities averts the costs of long-term care (US $80 to $150/day in 2009). Supportive IVR monitoring costs little after the initial outlay and is an effective way to support informal care-giving by family members, who want their elder relative to remain in the home for as long as possible (Mahoney et al., 2003).

IVR services are useful for less serious problems and monitoring chronic conditions. They cannot replace FTF intervention for serious problems.

Variations and Combinations of IVR Interventions

IVR systems provide a flexible platform for many therapeutic functions, including assessment and tailored feedback; as a stand-alone intervention or adjunct to FTF professional care; as a long-term monitoring and supportive intervention for chronic disorders that provides linkages to care; or as a reminder system to clients to attend appointments, take medications, or engage in scheduled "behavioral prescriptions." IVR systems can also perform practice management functions related to scheduling appointments, alerting clinic staff when clients need immediate attention (e.g., when violence or suicidal intentions are reported), and tracking the client base of a practice. Appendix 6 provides best practice guidelines for use of IVR systems in behavioral applications, based on our experience and the recommendations of Abu-Hasaballah et al. (2007).

Problems in Carrying Out IVR Interventions

IVR systems to should be firewalled and comply with relevant data protection requirements.

Despite the ease of use and low cost to callers, IVR systems entail ongoing financial costs and system management. Programming IVR software and producing output that can be used easily by busy providers requires programmer time and costs. An IVR system requires dedicated telephone lines and computers that are firewalled to protect client confidentiality and that satisfy HIPAA or other data protection requirements for health information systems. Ethical guidelines for IVR and other telehealth practices remain underdeveloped.

IVR systems usually provide clients with a toll-free number and a personal identification number to access their IVR data file at the start of calls, which is separated from identifying information. Telephone service can be interrupted, and staff alerts and a system back-up plan are needed. When IVR systems are used to make automated calls, client phone numbers and other contact information need to be updated regularly, and safeguards need to be in place so that the automated IVR calls are identified properly and not confused with telemarketing calls. See Abu-Hasaballah et al. (2007) for recommendations about these and other IVR implementation issues.

Multicultural Issues

The telephone is widely used worldwide and poses no obvious barriers in multicultural applications. IVR systems eliminate literacy concerns because there is nothing to read, although reading may be involved during training in some complex applications. Another benefit is that the voice recordings can be done in any language and by male or female actors of any age or ethnic origin. Callers can select their preferred language and gender. The capacity for such customization and consumer choice is a major advantage.

Older phones with a handset separate from the touch-tone keypad are easier to use than cell phones, which require callers to stop listening briefly when they enter responses (Abu-Hasaballah et al., 2007). Older adults with visual or motor impairments likely prefer or need a landline phone with a larger keypad.

4.2.3   Other Behavioral Health Cell Phone Applications

Description

As summarized in Table 7, in addition to IVR interventions, cell phones have been used in other ways to gather assessment information and deliver behavioral health interventions. Cell phone voice and Short Message Service (SMS) have been used, for example, to manage asthma symptoms and treatment regimen adherence (Holtz & Whitten, 2009) and to improve attendance at medical appointments (Koshy, Car, & Majeed, 2008). Typically, SMS approaches deliver short messages at preset or random intervals to participants' cell phones to reinforce health-related themes (e.g., diet and exercise, monitoring of personal air flow).

Mechanisms of Action

Cell phone applications function like other opportunistic interventions that seek to reach end users with messages that motivate, educate, and direct behavior. The mechanisms of action involved in efficacious IVR interventions generally apply to cell phone applications, which may have greater potential for yielding benefits because they can be used in the natural environment with high frequency and in highly personalized ways. When it comes to motivating and influencing people to modify behavior, cell phones have advantages over computers with respect to timing and context, in that "intervening at the right time and the right place increases the chances of getting results" (Fogg, 2009; p. 155). Unlike print materials and like IVR applications, cell phones can be used with high frequency over long intervals and are near-constant companions for most people. They have the added advantage of the use of video. They are thus perhaps the ideal extensive intervention platform to support stepped care. In addition to receiving behavior change messages, cell phone users can call for help in high-risk situations for resuming poor behavioral health practices or when they are experiencing distressing symptoms.

> Cell phone interventions allow more flexibility in timing and context than computer-based interventions.

Efficacy and Prognosis

Although more preliminary than for IVR studies as a whole, research indicates that cell phone voice and SMS interventions can help individuals implement positive changes and reduce adverse health-related outcomes. For example, a

Evaluation studies are less conclusive for cell phone and SMS than for IVR, but they also appear to improve quality of care and health outcomes.

review of studies from 1996 to 2007 showed that diabetes self-management interventions delivered by cell phone were efficacious with children and adults, typically as part of an overall program of care (Krishna & Boren, 2008). Improvements were found on measures of knowledge gained, behavior change, clinical improvement, and improved health status. For instance, 9 of 10 studies that measured glycated hemoglobin (HbA1c), a biological marker of blood sugar control, found significant improvements among recipients of cell phone interventions. Voice and text messages increased patient–provider and parent–child communication, as well as overall satisfaction with care. However, only one study used cell phones as a stand-alone intervention. The others included FTF clinic visits.

Another review evaluated whether cell phone voice and text messaging interventions improved health outcomes and processes of care (Krishna, Boren, & Balas, 2009). The 20 RCTs and 5 controlled studies involved 38,060 participants from 13 countries and covered 12 clinical specialties. Message frequency ranged from five a day for diabetes and smoking cessation to once a week for information and advice on how to counter barriers to maintaining regular physical activity. Significant improvements were found for medication adherence, asthma symptoms, HbA1c, stress levels, quit rates for smoking, and self-efficacy for appropriately dealing with specific health problems. Process improvements included fewer missed appointments and quicker diagnosis and treatment. These reviews showed that standard care could be enhanced with re-minders, disease monitoring, and management, and that education through cell phone voice and SMS improved health outcomes and care processes. Other SMS cell phone interventions yielded positive results for smoking cessation (Rodgers et al., 2005), diabetes self-management (Franklin, Wallet, Pagliari, & Greene, 2006), and weight loss (Patrick et al., 2009).

Variations and Combinations of Methods

Cell phones can be used to provide voice or text reminders in real time, e.g. for medication, diet, or exercise.

Like IVR systems, cell phones provide a flexible platform for potential thera-peutic functions and services, including use as a stand-alone assessment or intervention; as an adjunct to FTF professional care; or as a long-term monitor-ing and supportive intervention for chronic problems. Cell phones can deliver voice and text messages that prompt clients in real time to exercise, take medi-cation, or perform other scheduled behavioral prescriptions.

Problems in Carrying Out Cell Phone Applications

Cell phones are increasingly inexpensive and "smart" as they offer customized internet access. Their potential behavioral health applications are vast. However, as with IVR systems, challenges lie in programming assessment and interven-tion delivery via cell phone and in devising the computer interface and elec-tronic files. Another issue is ensuring that the resulting health applications are easy for end users to negotiate. Although cell phones are widely used for voice communication by all population segments, younger people are far more expe-rienced with cell phone texting and internet applications than many older adults.

Younger people remain more experienced with texting and internet cell phone applications.

Multicultural Issues

Cell phones have been widely adopted across racial, ethnic, and socioeco-nomic lines and can be personalized like no other technology. Whereas a "digital divide" exists for internet use between Whites and other ethnic and racial groups, in the United States, for example, strikingly similar high percentages of different groups use cell phones (e.g., 84%, 83%, and 89%, among US Whites, African Americans, and English-speaking Hispanics, respectively; Pew Internet & American Life Project, 2009). Use of internet services provided via cell phone has increased in recent years, especially among African Americans and English-speaking Hispanics. Given these trends and the rapid advances in cell phone technology that support internet access, cell phones may well become the most accessible platform for promoting behavior change, and their use deserves wider development and evaluation.

> The racial/ethnic gap seen with internet access has largely disappeared with respect to cell phone access.

4.2.4   High-Technology Treatment Modalities

Description
Computer-supported applications provide additional tools to reach large numbers of recipients with behavioral health interventions that can be tailored and directly marketed to consumers of services (Graham & Abrams, 2005). Although computer access and utilization lag behind cell phone adoption, as shown in Table 8, computer use, at least for email, has diffused to the great majority of the US population, and the sociodemographic characteristics of internet users are becoming less divergent.

> Computer applications support tailoring with less professional involvement than clinical care and can accommodate differences in literacy and learning style.

This is advantageous for behavioral health applications, which are summarized in Table 9. First, neither traditional public health nor clinical services have sufficient resources to address fully the public's health and MH/SU needs. Computer-supported programs that meld the two approaches can provide additional, sustainable, and complementary services to fill gaps in the continuum of care inside and outside of the health care system. Second, computer applications that take advantage of advances in information and health communication over the past 2 decades provide unprecedented opportunities to deliver tailored, theory-directed interventions to large numbers of people matched with their individual needs, resources, and readiness to change (Johnson et al., 2006; Prochaska et al., 1993). Third, computers, the internet, and other interactive health communication applications (e.g., mobile phones, interactive videos, hand-held computers or personal digital assistants [PDAs], CD-ROMs, and DVDs) allow practitioners to be more proactive in preventing, diagnosing, and treating behavioral health problems based on where people are in the change process. Fourth, multimedia interventions have audio features; can include graphics and videos, which lessen literacy concerns; and can address cultural issues and learning styles of diverse users.

> In addition to patient care functions, computer applications are useful for aiding provider decision-making and for practice management.

Advances in technologies have, in effect, offered both the means and the market for health-enhancing products that "fit" the lifestyle of many in the general public and overcome some challenges of reactive clinical interventions with limited population impact. As described next, computer applications have included internet-delivered interventions, which can be distributed widely much like print materials, as well as clinic- and web-based interactive, multimedia assessment and intervention programs. The options also include computerized "expert systems," which are employed to solve problems and aid

Table 8
Demographic Characteristics of Internet Users in the United States

Characteristic	% using the internet
Gender	
Women	74
Men	74
Age (in years)	
18–29	93
30–49	81
50–64	70
65+	38
Race/ethnicity	
White, non-Hispanic	76
Black, non-Hispanic	70
Hispanic*	64
Geography	
Suburban	77
Urban	74
Rural	70
Household income (annual US dollars)	
< $30,000	60
$30,000–$49,000	76
$50,000–$74,000	83
≥ $75,000	94
Education	
< High school	39
High school	63
Some college	87
College	94

Note. N = 2,258 adults, 18 years and older, including 565 cell phones; margin of error is ± 2%. *Hispanics include both English- and Spanish-speaking respondents. Reproduced from "Tracking Survey (November 30–December 27, 2009)," by Pew Internet & American Life Project, 2009, retrieved from http://www. pewinternet.org/Reports/2009/12-Wireless-Internet-Use.aspx. Copyright 2009 by Pew Internet & American Life Project.

Table 9
High-Technology Approaches for Behavioral Health Interventions

Internet applications
- Medium to high technology for end users and providers
- Supports tailoring and individual feedback, ongoing assessment
- Universal, selective, and indicated prevention
- Stand-alone or adjunct to professional care; self-monitoring, and self-management
- Broad reach to majority of population who have internet access
- End users access system by personal computer; providers set up and maintain hardware, software, and data files

Table 9
continued

- Private; convenient; no costs in addition to internet access; allows real-time interactions and reports; enhances sensitive reports; minimal user literacy required if material is written at the appropriate level and supplemented with graphics and audio
- Provider start-up costs high for hardware, software, programming, and management; for some projects, outsourcing may reduce provider costs
- End user must have internet access; persons in remote areas have limited access to FTF therapy but also may have higher costs and more difficulty gaining access to technology

Other electronic applications
- Medium to high technology for end users and providers
- Most applications support tailoring, individual feedback, and ongoing assessment
- Selective and indicated prevention
- Personal digital assistants, hand-held computers, interactive CDs, DVDs, and other electronic products can serve as stand-alone delivery channels or as adjuncts to more intense therapeutic encounters
- End users access system by personal computer or other electronic device; providers set up and maintain hardware and create, distribute, and update media (software, interactive DVD, etc.)
- Broad reach to majority of population with personal computers; convenient; low cost for users; can allow real-time interactions and reports; minimal user literacy required if material is written at the appropriate level and supplemented with graphics and audio
- Provider start-up costs lower than for internet applications, but still significant for hardware, software, programming, and management; media must be updated frequently to keep up with advances in technology; for some projects, outsourcing may reduce provider costs
- The digital divide for end users is shrinking, but it has not been eliminated; end users of limited means may not have access or may lack the most up-to-date technology to take full advantage of media features

Expert systems
- Medium to high technology for end users; high technology for providers
- Supports highest level of tailoring and individual feedback
- Selected and indicated prevention and maintenance
- Generally stand-alone but can be used as adjunct to other professional care
- Can be online or offline; also can be delivered by cell phone or landline or mailed to the end user's home to broaden reach; minimal user literacy required at higher levels of technology (graphics and audio)
- Development can be costly; time-consuming for the experts involved; all possible combinations of end-user responses must be addressed during development
- Lower technology versions that increase access do not provide feedback in real time; higher technology versions with more features and lower literacy requirements are less accessible due to cost for end users

Note. FTF = face-to-face.

real-life decision-making that normally would require specialist consultation (Negotia, 1985). These technology-driven intervention tools and channels may be used alone or in combination with FTF services.

Internet Applications: The internet is particularly useful for delivering health communications that utilize the economics of mass media and, at the same time, have the capacity to generate interventions that address individuals' needs based on responses to brief assessments, preprogrammed algorithms, and decision rules (Abrams & Emmons, 1997). Interventions that target individuals at risk at the population level can be used to facilitate and maintain behavior change. The internet is optimal for implementing real-time, individualized communication messages and intervention strategies because of its flexibility and sustainability. Once developed and implemented, such "e-Health" applications possess the ability to reach a large number of end users at relatively low cost as compared with traditional, offline interventions (Ahern, 2007).

Other Personal Computer Applications: The PC in its many forms has become a delivery channel of health information for the public and providers alike. For example, physicians use handheld computers or PDAs to assist them with making diagnoses and prescribing medications for patients. Clients can use PDAs to record real-time data regarding their thoughts and behaviors, thereby reducing potential forgetting and biased recall.

Clinical assessment data can also be recorded easily on a PC, and records can be downloaded into databases for analysis and application. PC-supported applications allow for standardized presentation and collection of information, normative and tailored feedback based on individual needs and assessment responses, provision of individualized interventions to large numbers of people, and access and sustainability over time. A case in point is the computerized version of the Addiction Severity Index (ASI), which is a psychometrically sound, widely adopted, interview-based assessment. Because valid FTF administration requires extensive interviewer training, Budman (2000) developed a multimedia computer-administered version that uses virtual interviewers, provides information, and escorts users through the program. The computerized version has demonstrated similar psychometric properties to live administration by a skilled clinician.

> **Computerized versions of validated assessments often show similar psychometric properties to FTF administration at much lower cost.**

Computer software has the capacity to deliver intervention messages and to change unhealthy behaviors while reducing therapist contact time and containing costs. For example, Bickel and colleagues (Bickel, Marsch, Buchhalter, & Badger, 2008) developed and evaluated an interactive, computerized behavioral intervention for opioid-dependent outpatients based on the community reinforcement approach (CRA) plus a voucher-based contingency management model. The computer-delivered intervention was compared in an RCT with a therapist-delivered CRA intervention plus vouchers and a standard-care treatment condition. The computer- and therapist-delivered interventions resulted in similar positive changes in substance-related outcomes that were significantly greater than the standard treatment group. The computer version offered greater dissemination potential of the evidence-based CRA plus vouchers treatment and ensured treatment fidelity. The text box provides another example of a very brief computerized intervention guided by the TTM to increase condom use among patients seen in a busy urban public clinic for sexually transmitted diseases (STDs).

Computerized Risk Reduction Intervention in a Public Clinic for Sexually Transmitted Diseases

Counseling for risk reduction can change sexual risk behaviors and prevent new sexually transmitted diseases (STDs), and clinic visits for acute STD care may be the only opportunity to promote risk reduction in some persons at increased risk. However, provision of STD prevention counseling may be constrained by competing clinical priorities in busy public STD clinics. To address this service delivery challenge, Grimley and Hook (2009) developed and evaluated a single, brief (15-minute), theory-based, computerized intervention designed to increase condom use with a main or steady sexual partner and to reduce new cases of infection by *Neisseria gonorrhoeae* and *Chlamydia trachomatis*.

Predominately lower income, African-American patients (*N* = 430) were recruited while waiting for clinical care in an urban STD clinic. Random assignment to a transtheoretical model (TTM)-based intervention or control condition was stratified by gender, sexual orientation, and baseline stage of change for condom use based on initial computer assessment. The intervention group then received individualized stage-matched behavioral messages and feedback based on TTM constructs. Intervention messages simultaneously appeared on the computer screen and were heard by users through headphones to limit literacy concerns while protecting privacy. The control group interacted with a 15-minute, computerized health risk assessment without receiving intervention messages. Participants returned to the clinic at 6 months and were reassessed on stage of change for consistent (100%) condom use. Biological specimens were also collected.

At 6 months, brief intervention recipients were more likely to report condom use 100% of the time with a main partner in the preceding 2 months compared with controls (*p* = .03). No significant gender differences were found. The overall STD rates at 6 months for the intervention and control groups were 6% and 13%, respectively. Compared with baseline STD prevalence, the difference in proportions of STD rates decreased 22% for the intervention group versus 3% for the control group from baseline to 6 months (*p* = .04).

The study showed that a single, brief, interactive, computer-delivered intervention at a routine clinic visit increased consistent condom use and reduced STDs without burdening clinic staff or interfering with clinical care. Such interventions based on a person's readiness for changing risk behaviors are potentially cost-effective and sustainable and can benefit STD clinic patients if thoughtfully integrated with other activities during the visit.

Practitioners interested in such computer applications can use newly developed, innovative software developed by Grimley and colleagues (available from author D.M.G.). These researchers have developed software that provides interfaces for building Web 2.0 aware rich-content assessments with individualized interventions delivered via the internet and smartphones, and it has three built-in security systems. What makes this software "engine" unique is that it can be applied to any physical or MH/SU condition, customized to support different behavior change theories and models, and it can do this with no reconfiguration of the existing software. No new code needs to be written because all assessments, intervention messages, algorithms, and decision rules have been placed outside of the software itself. The software is deployed using another common, inexpensive software called "software as a service." The system, designed and developed with US National Institutes of Health (NIH)

"Software as a Service" can reduce costs by allowing practitioners to rent a needed program for only the time or number of uses needed.

funding, is being employed in an internet-delivered intervention that targets reproductive health. It is being evaluated through a double-blind RCT with adolescent and young adult females ages 14-25 recruited from three clinics in the southeastern United States.

Expert Systems: Considered a subfield of artificial intelligence, expert or knowledge systems are software programmed to solve problems and make decisions in real-life situations, e.g., to help a physician diagnose diseases based on patients' symptoms. Expert systems reason with domain-specific "deep" knowledge that is symbolic and numerical and use domain-specific methods that are plausible, heuristic, and experience-based to solve problems and quickly arrive at optimal solutions. Expert systems also use algorithms, scoring systems, and decision rules referred to as "surface" knowledge (Barr, Cohen, & Feigenbaum, 1989).

Many so-called expert systems used in preventive health care today rely heavily on surface knowledge and are rule-based systems that use conditional sentences relating statements of facts with one another (Buchanan & Duda, 1982). Relatively few use deep knowledge, which reflects dynamic theories and principles of behavior change. Further advances in application will depend on undergirding the systems with well-specified theories and principles.

A Home-Based Expert System Intervention to Promote Hypertensive Medication Adherence Among Patients in Pre-Action Stages of Change

Johnson and colleagues (2006) developed and evaluated a home-based expert system intervention based on the transtheoretical model (TTM) to increase proper hypertension medication use among US health maintenance organization (HMO) patients (*N* = 1,227) who participated by mail. Interrelationships among the model's core constructs (e.g., stages and processes of change) provided the deep knowledge for generating the tailored interventions, and research findings and experience-based heuristics provided the surface knowledge for rule-based decision-making.

Nonadhering patients in pre-action stages of change were recruited by mail and randomized to intervention or control conditions. The intervention group received by mail three computerized TTM-based printouts based on assessment responses also collected by mail at baseline, 3, and 6 months. The printouts included strategies related to the model's four constructs, normative data regarding how participants compared with others in the same stage, ipsative comparisons with their own assessments from one point to the next, and a stage-matched manual with behavioral recommendations. Follow-up data were collected at 12 and 18 months. Control participants completed the assessments by mail at baseline and at 6, 12, and 18 months.

Although the two groups did not differ at 6 months, the treatment group reported significantly better medication adherence than the control group at the 12- and 18-month follow-ups. While the absence of objective adherence checks is a limitation, the study found apparent sustained therapeutic effects using an expert system with a large HMO patient sample in the pre-action stages of change that could be implemented by mail. The study supported the utility of expert systems as an alternative to clinic-based care for patients who were not seeking help and who were not highly motivated to change an important health behavior.

Expert systems can be online or offline and have been developed for use with different populations for diverse behaviors including smoking cessation (Prochaska et al., 1993), STD/HIV prevention (Grimley & Hook, 2009), and hypertension medication adherence (Johnson et al., 2006), to name a few. Decision rules allow for individualized information to be generated for the end user, similar to a human interaction, but at lower cost and with broader reach (Grimley & Hook, 2009). The text box describes an expert system application to promote medication adherence among hypertensive patients in pre-action stages of change (Johnson et al., 2006).

"Expert systems" allow for tailoring of interactions at a lower cost and with broader reach than FTF interventions.

Efficacy and Prognosis

There is evidence that internet-delivered interventions accurately communicate feedback based on the end user's specific needs and effectively change health risk behaviors. A review of 85 RCTs (Webb, Joseph, Yardley, & Michie, 2010; total $N = 43{,}236$) found a small but significant overall effect size ($d = .16$, 95% CI = .09, .23). Interventions employing theory more extensively ($p = .049$) or employing a greater number of change techniques ($p < .01$) were relatively more effective.

Internet-based and other computer-delivered interventions have shown varying degrees of efficacy. For example, studies comparing the efficacy of programs delivered over the internet versus those delivered FTF have shown that the two delivery channels lead to similar, clinically meaningful results (Wantland et al., 2004). Comparable findings have been reported for other computer-delivered interventions for a variety of behavioral health problems, including alcohol use among heavy-drinking college students (Butler & Correia, 2009), co-occurring depression and alcohol/cannabis use among adults (Kay-Lambkin et al., 2009), and symptoms of anxiety disorders (Kenardy et al., 2003). For example, in a multicenter, international RCT of CBT for panic disorder (Kenardy et al., 2003), at the end of treatment and at 6 months postintervention, a 12-session FTF CBT condition and a 6-session CBT plus PDA condition were similarly efficacious, and both resulted in better improvements than a control condition. Similar to Bickel et al. (2008), this study showed that PDAs can reduce therapist contact time without reducing treatment benefits. Noar et al. (2009) conducted a meta-analysis of 12 RCTs that evaluated computer-based HIV prevention interventions designed to increase condom use with various at-risk populations ($N = 4{,}639$). The overall mean weighted effect size for condom use was $d = 0.259$ (95% CI = 0.201, 0.317; $Z = 8.74$, $p < .001$), demonstrating a significant impact of the computer-based interventions that was similar to previously observed effect sizes for interventions delivered by human facilitators. Interventions were more efficacious when they were gender-based, provided individualized tailoring, used the TTM, and had more sessions. The findings strongly supported the use of computerized technology-based intervention programs for HIV prevention and control.

Internet-based and other computer-delivered interventions have shown varying degrees of efficacy.

Variations and Combinations of High-Technology Interventions

Computerized and internet-based interventions, cell phones, interactive CD-ROMs, videos, and other electronic products have the capacity to serve as stand-alone delivery channels or as adjuncts to FTF therapeutic encounters. This is useful because not all clients need the same type or intensity of intervention.

Technology-delivered interventions are a useful addition to the stepped care model of service delivery.

Technology-delivered interventions have an important role in the continuum of care and are useful in a stepped care model of care (Sobell & Sobell, 2000) .

Another use of computerized assessment is to collect information on provider practice patterns in real-time. The American Psychological Association developed PracticeNet for this purpose (see https://www.apapracticenet.net/introduction.asp) and has used it to monitor the practices of psychologists and to assess the impact on clinical presentations of disasters such as the 9/11 terrorist attack on the New York World Trade Center. Such applications blur lines between research and practice and can support the detection of practice trends and new or rare phenomena, thus enabling services and associated research to be redirected quickly.

Problems with Carrying Out High-Technology Interventions

Despite the many advantages associated with high-technology interventions, the "digital divide" in the availability and adoption of computer technology remains a problem for practitioners attempting to reach underserved populations. However, the divide is slowly closing; cell phone use has been adopted rapidly by diverse populations; and cell phones function more and more as portable computers that offer email, internet, and web access.

The digital divide is shrinking, but access still is not universal. Some individuals simply prefer human interaction.

Not everyone will prefer interacting with electronic interventions due to the lack of human contact. Such applications cannot capitalize on the therapeutic benefits of personal contact, nor can they make use of nonverbal communication (Taylor & Luce, 2003). Nevertheless, when clinicians use such tools as adjuncts to FTF interventions, the electronic component often comes to be treated like a person by clients, who may view computers as having personalities and respond to them in ways similar to their approaches to human encounters (Budman, 2000).

Other potential problems are more technical or practical. For example, depending on the level of tailoring (number of variables being tailored on), the development of intervention messages and strategies based on all possible combinations of responses can be labor-intensive. Start-up costs can be fairly substantial. Nevertheless, web-based programs can be widely diffused, are sustainable, and can be made available to consumers online. This usually offsets the initial start-up costs. However, not all behavior change applications online are valid, and many legitimate applications are generic. A recent content analysis of 497 consumer-oriented health websites (Suggs & McIntyre, 2007) showed that 406 provided generic content only, 41 provided personalized information, 37 were targeted interventions to specific groups, and only 13 provided tailored information. Practitioners need to inform the people they serve that many online health applications have been designed (accurately or not) for the general public's use and do not take into account individual characteristics that are basic to facilitating behavioral health.

Many online health applications are designed generically and do not address individual characteristics that may be important for effective care.

Another limitation is that few studies have reported in sufficient detail on the underlying theoretical framework used to develop interventions. Different theories and models may be more suitable to specific health behaviors (e.g., behavioral economics for addictive behaviors), and certain delivery channels may provide a better "fit" for different health behaviors.

Internet-delivered treatment programs attract groups that have computer access and literacy, which has resulted in sampling biases in the research base.

This situation is improving with the widespread use of cell phones by more diverse populations who have daily access to the web. Even among internet users, attrition has been relatively high for internet behavioral treatment programs if end users were not part of a research study with a closed website (Christensen, Griffiths, & Farrer, 2009). Furthermore, the technology market is constantly changing, and behavioral health applications risk lagging behind consumer preferences in technologies and becoming dated.

Internet-based programs attract groups with computer access, and programs must keep up with ever-changing technologies to remain relevant.

Multicultural Issues

Despite the barriers discussed above, high-technology behavioral health applications have nearly unlimited capacity to reach and cover the population in all its diversity. Providing health and MH/SU services to everyone is an equity value at the core of public health practice. Clinical care cannot achieve equitable service delivery without public health and behavioral health programs. As in all other technological applications, the influence of culture must be considered when designing, delivering, and evaluating web-based software and other behavioral health intervention programs.

4.3 Unresolved Issues and Future Directions

Despite the breadth of applications discussed in this chapter, behavioral health applications that involve phone and computer technology are in their infancy as a practice and a science. To date, the TTM is the only theoretical perspective that has been used to any extent to guide tailored interventions. It has fared reasonably well, although it has limitations. Other theories such as behavioral economics are firmly established in guiding FTF interventions, but technological applications are only now being developed (Bickel et al., 2008). Further development of behavior change theories generally, and evidence-based interventions using phone and computer technology specifically, will be important for advancing the population impact of behavioral health services.

Tailored interventions have relied heavily on the transtheoretical model. However, incremental benefits of exhaustive tailoring have not been well researched.

Another important undecided issue is the extent to which gains in outcomes are accrued with greater individualization and tailoring of interventions. Available evidence on this point is mixed in the FTF efficacy research literature (e.g., Murphy et al., 2004), and further research is needed. Some degree of personalization based on individual information seems beneficial in combination with normative health-related information and messages, but whether exhaustive personalization and tailoring further improve outcomes remains unclear.

As a whole, media- and technology-based interventions have been developed and evaluated to a greater degree for health-related behaviors (e.g., diabetes, addictive behaviors, medication adherence, HIV risk reduction) than for mental health disorders. Work on the latter applications is growing and applications developed to date have shown initial success. However, a gap remains in applications involving mental health research and practice compared with health behaviors.

Finally, to reap the full potential population impact of using media and technology to extend the scope of practice, the various approaches discussed in

Technology and clinical methods should be used in combination to form a continuum of care.

this chapter need to be assembled along with clinical and public health methods to form an effective continuum of care. The research agenda that flows from combining clinical, behavioral health, and public health strategies into an integrated continuum of care is complex, as epitomized by social ecological models of behavior change (see Figure 5). Combination strategies and tactics in a system of care should rest on studies of the efficacy and effectiveness of individual components. In several areas of application, the necessary evidence base is available or growing rapidly; in others, it is nascent.

Services for real-world health and behavioral health problems always need and benefit from innovation and improvements, and the implementation of new approaches often understandably outpaces the evidence base. In Chapter 5, we offer a case vignette that puts many of the pieces discussed in this chapter together in a system of care for HIV/AIDS prevention and treatment in a disadvantaged rural community. This is based on a real clinic in our home state of Alabama. We hope it inspires readers as has it us to take some of the single interventions covered in this chapter and consider how to use them in concert to develop a continuum of care for serious health and behavioral health problems that spans the prevention and treatment service sectors shown in Figure 1.

5

Case Vignette

As intervention options have expanded beyond individual psychotherapy, roles for doctoral level mental health professionals have expanded as well. Today's doctoral professionals often help design, implement, and evaluate behavioral health service delivery systems that offer a range of low- to high-intensity services. They may work in for-profit MCO behavioral health carve-outs, in primary care medical clinics, or in under-resourced community clinics that serve disadvantaged groups. They may write proposals to obtain funding for innovative MH/SU programs and may oversee program implementation and staff training. In an expanded system of care that reaches from the clinic into the community, subdoctoral staff members or paraprofessionals often do the bulk of direct service delivery, while doctoral professionals reserve their time for complex cases and quality-assurance functions.

A Day at a Nonprofit Integrative "One-Stop-Shop" Clinic for Persons Living with HIV/AIDS in Rural Alabama

To illustrate contemporary approaches to providing integrated behavioral health care in an under-resourced rural setting, we asked our colleague Cathy A. Simpson, PhD, to describe a typical day in her work at a small clinic in rural Alabama that provides medical and behavioral health services to persons living with HIV/AIDS. Dr. Simpson is a licensed clinical psychologist who has had a significant role in designing, implementing, and evaluating a multilevel approach to integrated behavioral health care at a non-profit AIDS service organization that is described in the text box. Dr. Simpson is in independent practice and contracts her services to the Health Services Center, Inc. (HSC). She also is a part-time associate professor in the School of Public Health at the nearby University of Alabama at Birmingham. We believe her work at HSC exemplifies new roles and opportunities for doctoral psychologists educated as scientist–practitioners and that the behavioral health services offered at HSC illustrate how the tools of clinical and public health practice can be woven together to provide seamless care for disadvantaged persons living with HIV/ AIDS. The example describes a typical day of agency-wide service provision. Client and staff characteristics have been modified to protect individual confidentiality, but the services described are real. We join the staff as they begin their work day at the main HSC facility in Hobson City, Alabama.

8:00 a.m. The medical clinic opens. The clinic opens and patients with appointments begin to be seen for routine HIV-related medical care services.

Integrative "One-Stop-Shop" Care for Persons Living With HIV/AIDS

The Health Services Center, Inc. (HSC) is a nonprofit, community-based organization that serves a 14-county, 9,000-square-mile area in northeast Alabama. The service area lies in the southeastern United States, which has rising HIV incidence and prevalence rates, particularly among people of color. The agency was founded in 1987 by Barbara J. Hanna, MD, who has been its Medical Director since inception. HSC operates a primary facility in Hobson City, Alabama, and four satellite clinics with vans to transport staff and patients between locations. In addition to the typical barriers encountered to health care access, the HSC catchment area is marked by underserved populations and includes barriers to health care such as poverty, low literacy, and lack of access to educational services; long travel distances to medical and mental health services; and mistrust of medical and social services systems.

HSC serves approximately 450 clients annually through direct medical services and provides substance abuse treatment and prevention services, as well as HIV and hepatitis prevention services to another 5,000 members of the local communities annually. The organization has a full-time staff of about 40, including medical and mental health professionals, clinical social workers, health education specialists, other health behavior professionals, and paraprofessionals. The organization contracts with a clinical psychologist to evaluate program outcomes.

HSC strives to lower the threshold to clinical care through use of a one-stop-shop model. Functionally, this approach seeks to make available a menu of service options for medical clients and other community members who have varying levels of HIV-related risk and behavior change needs. These needs include ongoing medical management, intensive medical and psychosocial case management, targeted prevention services, and brief outreach and testing services. In addition to increasing client and community access to care, the one-stop-shop approach is a cost-effective means of integrating services that support prevention and health behavior change with primary medical and mental health and substance use (MH/SU) services.

The scheduled medical case load for the day is 57 patients. While waiting to see the physician or a nurse practitioner, patients are seated in a comfortable waiting area where local churches and community groups (e.g., sororities, Rotary Clubs) have provided lunch and light refreshments. During this time, patients have access to printed materials promoting a range of health behaviors, including safer sex and alcohol and drug education. Additional materials focus on cardiovascular health, diabetes management, and family issues such as domestic violence and how to talk to teenagers about behavioral health issues. A television in the waiting area provides a looping video series about health and preventive behaviors. Today, the video is "Safe in the City," a CDC-produced public health series about reducing HIV risk behaviors for sexually active adults.

9:00 a.m. Taking advantage of waiting time. As clients sign in for their appointments, Angela, the clinic receptionist, is alerted by the computerized medical information system concerning which patients need a case management visit to assess for psychosocial needs and which ones need a brief substance use or mental health screening. These screenings are conducted quickly, and clients with risk factors are routed for additional assessment and consultation while they wait for their medical appointment. The typical waiting time for a medical appointment is 30 to 45 minutes, and most screenings and video health promotion can be conducted during this anticipated "downtime."

10:00 a.m. Brief street outreach services. While medical staff members are conducting scheduled health visits, other HSC staff members are working in the community to provide brief street outreach and prevention messages. Today, lead outreach worker James is conducting outreach at a local barbershop for the Project REAL program. While talking with customers about preventive behaviors and the importance of health screenings, James encounters two men who are interested in receiving an HIV test. Neither of the men knows his HIV status or has ever considered himself at risk, but now they are not so sure. Testing, which James explains is quick and confidential, sounds like a good option. James arranges immediate rapid oral HIV testing and counseling for both men in a private room in the back of the shop.

11:00 a.m. Screening, brief counseling, and referral; midpoint of medical service delivery for the day. At the main clinic, medical service delivery continues. Monica, a mother of two in her mid-30s, meets with her physician, Dr. Smith. The medical information system alerts Dr. Smith that Monica is due for a quarterly screening for nutrition and an annual dietary assessment. Dr. Smith also takes a moment to review the substance use and mental health screenings that Monica completed while waiting for the appointment. Based on Monica's body mass index and the results of her dietary assessment, Dr. Smith conducts brief counseling on the importance of physical activity and weight management and refers Monica to the onsite nutritionist for sample menus. Monica also is informed about a new clinic program focused on increasing physical activity and reducing cardiovascular risk. Monica agrees to participate and will receive weekly phone calls from a clinic paraprofessional to assist her in charting her progress. As Monica takes her prescriptions and checks out with the receptionist, the medical information system reminds the receptionist to schedule Monica for a brief visit with a case manager to evaluate her physical activity progress before her next appointment with Dr. Smith.

12:00 p.m. Extending support to caregivers. While waiting with his wife for her medical appointment, Chester, a middle-aged teacher, is approached by Dr. Jones, a contracted psychologist at the clinic. Dr. Jones and two assistant counselors are offering groups for caregivers and family members of persons living with HIV. Chester is initially skeptical as his schedule already is filled with work, appointments, and childcare duties. Dr. Jones points out that the group is meeting during patient clinic appointment times when Chester typically would already be at the clinic. Chester agrees to participate and spends the next half hour talking with other spouses and family members of patients about issues such as discussing HIV disease with their children, working through depression and anxiety, and incorporating relaxation and physical activity into daily routines. Although his participation is relatively short, Chester leaves the clinic feeling more connected with the community. He also has a list of websites for caregivers, a hotline number, and the name of a clinic mental health counselor working with Dr. Jones who can provide additional assistance if needed.

1:00 p.m. Preparing for behavior change. At the barbershop, James's outreach efforts have been very successful for the day. Both men who completed quick oral HIV testing were negative for HIV, and both were provided with safer sex kits and one-on-one information about ways to reduce risks. One of the men, Alberto, is concerned about the risks posed by his current behaviors; however, he is ambivalent about making any major life changes just yet. James refers Alberto to an ongoing HSC prevention program called PEaPLE First. The program works with active substance users who are at risk of contracting HIV disease or viral hepatitis. When Alberto attends his first session, he finds that the program does not insist that he change everything all at once. Instead, the case manager talks with Alberto and others in the group about their specific risks and asks them about areas in which they could begin making small changes toward safer behaviors. This approach seems different to Alberto, more like the real world than some of the all-or-nothing treatment programs he has been to before. He decides to set two initial goals: (1) reducing his number of sexual partners; and (2) getting tested for HIV every 3 months. These sound to Alberto like things he might be able to do. Maybe later he'll try some of the other risk reduction strategies as well. At the end of the session, the group leader refers Alberto to the HSC medical clinic for a hepatitis screening.

2:00 p.m. Maintenance and self-monitoring. Carla, a long-time HSC patient in her mid-40s, picks up her cell phone and calls a toll-free number for the clinic. This is not a scheduled appointment day for Carla, nor is she seeking any direct medical services. Rather, Carla is participating in a new "telehealth" program at the clinic that allows her to self-monitor different health behaviors each day by phone, using a confidential, computerized IVR system. The phone rings, she is prompted to enter her personal identification number, and then a recorded voice asks her to use telephone keys to report on different health behaviors from the day before. For example, did she take her medications as prescribed, did she drink alcohol, and what were her mood states? Carla initially agreed to participate in the call-in program because she thought it sounded sort of interesting, and she could get a small gift card for trying out the system. One of the psychologists at the clinic suggested that she might enjoy the system and find it helpful after she got used to it. Now she calls daily because she finds that tracking her behavior each day and getting weekly reports from the system on how she's doing helps her to remember to take her HIV medication. She suspects tracking her mood daily also has helped her to be more in touch with some of the issues that have been making medication adherence difficult. The call takes about 3 minutes, and then she turns back to her computer at work to finish a project.

3:00 p.m. Substance abuse treatment. HSC's Behavioral Day Treatment for substance abuse, held in a nearby rented office, is ending for the day. The program is voluntary and provides clients with an intensive outpatient approach to substance abuse treatment that is based on community reinforcement principles and focuses on skills building, goal-setting, and learning to engage in substance-free leisure activities. Dan, a retired plumber, is particularly pleased today. He has achieved 100% of his goals for the week. In addition to the personal satisfaction of achieving the goals, he receives a small voucher that he can use to buy some much-needed toiletries and personal items. He is pleased as well because today was the twice-weekly attendance raffle, and he won a shaving kit. He looks at his watch and finds he has just enough time for the clinic van to take him to the main clinic for his consult with the nutritionist about his cholesterol screening.

4:00 p.m. Evaluation and follow-up. The day is winding down at HSC. Adherence specialists are reviewing the daily electronic notes and compiling a list of clients who might benefit from additional services or screenings. They are making preliminary individualized plans to discuss with those clients for their approval and engagement. The adherence specialists also note clients who did not attend scheduled appointments. They create a list to call the following day to set up make-up appointments for medical or MH/SU services and for discussion of ways to make visits easier for clients to attend. A clinical psychologist, contracted by HSC to evaluate the successes of and barriers to its programs, is reviewing the daily program data and compiling reports and suggestions for the clinic staff.

5:00 p.m. Preparation for additional services. The medical staff, mental health staff, and case managers close the clinic for the day, and on-call employees for the evening are identified. A brief meeting is held regarding two new programs. One focuses on increasing outreach and knowledge of HIV services for women, and the other aims to increase patient adherence to medical care, such as attendance at appointments and continued contact with case managers. Notes from different disciplines are compared, and the staff agrees on a 2-week work plan.

Note. The programs and services described in the vignette were variously supported in part by funding from the US Department of Health and Human Services – Ryan White Programs; US Substance Abuse and Mental Health Services Administration/Centers for Substance Abuse Treatment (SAMHSA/CSAT) – Targeted Capacity Expansion Grants Program; SAMHSA/Centers for Substance Abuse Prevention – Minority AIDS Council Initiative; US Centers for Disease Control and Prevention; National Institute on Drug Abuse grant no. 5R21DA21524; and local foundations.

6

Further Reading

Glanz, K., Rimer, B. K., & Viswanath, K. (Eds.) (2008). *Health behavior and health education* (4th ed.). San Francisco: Jossey-Bass.

This classic text summarizes and critiques an array of health behavior theories and includes evidence from the research literature.

Institute of Medicine (2003). *Who will keep the public healthy? Educating public health professionals for the 21st century.* Washington, DC: National Academies Press.

This volume provides an overview of past and present public health education and offers a road map for improvement and expansion.

Institute of Medicine (2006). *Improving the quality of health care for mental and substance-use conditions.* Washington, D.C.: National Academies Press.

This volume in the *Quality Chasm Series* assesses the state of quality of care in the de-facto mental health/substance abuse treatment system and proposes an agenda for improvement.

Madden, G. J., & Bickel, W. K. (Eds.) (2010). *Impulsivity: The behavioral and neurological science of discounting.* Washington, D.C.: APA Books.

This edited book provides a comprehensive overview of modern theory and research on impulsivity (delay discounting in particular) and includes chapters by leading researchers.

National Cancer Institute (2001). *Making health communication programs work.* Bethesda, MD: NCI/National Institutes of Health/US Department of Health and Human Services. Available at: http://www.cancer.gov/pinkbook.

This "how-to" guide, available at no charge from the NCI website, provides step-by-step planning tips and summaries of useful health communication theories and practices.

National Cancer Institute (2003). *Theory at a glance: A guide for health promotion Practice* (2nd ed.). US Department of Health and Human Services, NIH Publication No. 05-3896. Available at: http://www.cancer.gov/PDF/481f5d53-63df-41bc-bfaf-5aa48ee1da4d/TAAG3.pdf.

This brief user's guide to health behavior theory is available at no charge from the NCI website and offers brief summaries and examples of the most widely employed theories.

National Institute on Alcohol Abuse and Alcoholism (2005). *Helping patients who drink too much: A clinician's guide.* Rockville, MD: NIAAA/National Institutes of Health/US Department of Health and Human Services. Available at: http://pubs.niaaa.nih.gov/publications/Practitioner/CliniciansGuide2005/clinicians_guide.htm.

This free online kit offers tools for screening, brief intervention, and referral to treatment by primary care providers. Background and rationale for routine screening are described.

National Institutes of Health (2009). *NIH science of behavior change meeting summary.* Bethesda, MD: NIH/US Department of Health and Human Services. Available at: http://nihroadmap.nih.gov/documents/SOBC_Meeting_Summary_2009.pdf.

This conference summary articulates a roadmap for NIH aimed at promoting an expanded agenda for behavior change research that goes beyond clinical strategies to include public health strategies.

Prochaska, J. O., Norcross, J. C., & DiClemente, C. C. (1994). *Changing for good.* New York: William Morrow.

This book is written for lay-persons who are attempting to change risky or unhealthful behaviors or want to learn more about the change process. Useful examples of everyday situations and problems encountered are provided.

Tucker, J. A., Phillips, M. M., Murphy, J. G., & Raczynski, J. M. (2004). Behavioral epidemiology and health psychology. In R. G. Frank, A. Baum, & J. Wallander (Eds.), *Models and perspectives in health psychology* (pp. 435-464) (Vol. 3, *Handbook of Clinical Health Psychology*). Washington, DC: APA Books.

This chapter from the 3-volume APA series on clinical health psychology summarizes the behavioral epidemiology of mental health/substance use disorders and patterns of care-seeking from a population perspective.

Weinrech, N. K. (1999). *Hands on social marketing: A step-by-step guide.* Sage Publications: Thousand Oaks, CA.

This textbook provides background information, a planning guide, and sample forms for use in the implementation of social marketing campaigns.

WHO World Mental Health Survey Consortium (2004). Prevalence, severity, and unmet need for treatment of mental disorders in the World Health Organization Mental Health Surveys. *Journal of the American Medical Association, 291*, 2581-2590.

Comprehensive mental health data are reported from the WHO's World Mental Health Survey Initiative, which sampled 8 developed and 6 less developed national populations.

Wright, K., Sparks, L., & O'Hair, D. (2007). *Health communication in the 21st century.* Malden, MA: Blackwell.

This textbook offers a thorough introduction to health communication issues, theories, and practices and includes examples and case studies.

7

References

Abrams, D. B., & Emmons, K. M. (1997). Health behavior and health education: The past, present, and future. In K. Glanz., B. K. Rimer, & F. M. Lewis (Eds.), *Health behavior and health education: Theory, research, and practice* (pp. 453–478). San Francisco, CA: Jossey-Bass.

Abu-Hasaballah, K., James, A., & Aseltine, R. H., Jr. (2007). Lessons and pitfalls of interactive voice response in medical research. *Contemporary Clinical Trials, 28,* 593–602.

Ahern, D. K. (2007). Challenges and opportunities of eHealth research. *American Journal of Preventive Medicine, 32* (Supp. 1), S75–S82.

Ainslie, G. (1975). Specious reward: A behavioral theory of impulsiveness and impulse control. *Psychological Bulletin, 82,* 463–509.

Ajzen, I. (1985). From intentions to actions: A theory of planned behavior. In J. Kuhl & J. Beckmann (Eds.), *Action-control: From cognition to behavior* (pp. 11–39). Heidelberg: Springer.

American Psychological Association (2010). The Patient Protection and Affordable Care Act: New protections and opportunities for practicing psychologists. Retrieved from http://www.apapracticecentral.org/advocacy/reform/patient-protection.aspx

Bandura, A. (1977). Self-efficacy: Toward a unifying theory of behavioral change. *Psychological Review, 84,* 191–215.

Bandura, A. (1986). *Social foundation of thought and action: A social cognitive theory.* Englewood Cliffs, NJ: Prentice Hall.

Barr, A. B., Cohen, P. R., & Feigenbaum, E. A. (1989). *The handbook of artificial intelligence* (Vol. 4). Reading, MA: Addison Wesley.

Barta, W. D., Portnoy, D. B., Kiene, S. M., Tennan, H., Abu-Hasaballah, K. S., & Ferrer, R. (2008). A daily process investigation of alcohol-involved sexual risk behavior among economically disadvantaged problem drinkers living with HIV/AIDS. *AIDS and Behavior, 12,* 729–740.

Bickel, W. K., & Marsch, L. A. (2000). Toward a behavioral economic understanding of drug dependence: Delay discounting processes. *Addiction, 96,* 73–86.

Bickel, W. K., Marsch, L. A., Buchhalter, A. R., & Badger, G. J. (2008). Computerized behavior therapy for opioid-dependent outpatients: A randomized controlled trial. *Experimental and Clinical Psychopharmacology, 16,* 132–143.

Bickel, W. K., & Vuchinich, R. E. (Eds.). (2003). *Reframing health behavior change with behavioral economics.* Mahwah, NJ: Lawrence Erlbaum Associates.

Biener, L., & Abrams, D. (1991). The Contemplation Ladder: Validation of a measure of readiness to consider smoking cessation. *Health Psychology, 10,* 360–365.

Breslin, F. C., Sobell, L. C., Sobell, M. B., & Agrawal, S. (2000). A comparison of a brief and long version of the Situational Confidence Questionnaire. *Behaviour Research and Therapy, 38,* 1211–1220.

Buchanan, B. G., & Duda, R. O. (1982*). Principles of rule-based expert systems.* Technical Report: CS-TR-82-926. Stanford, CA: Stanford University Press.

Budman, S. H. (2000). Behavioral health care dot.com and beyond: Computer-mediated communication in mental health and substance abuse treatment. *American Psychologist, 55,* 1290–1300.

Butler, L. H., & Correia, C. J. (2009). Brief alcohol intervention with college student drinkers: Face-to-face versus computerized feedback. *Psychology of Addictive Behaviors, 23,* 163–167.

Chapman, G. B., & Johnson, E. J. (1995). Preference reversals in monetary and life expectancy evaluations. *Organizational Behavior and Human Decision Processes, 65,* 300–317.

Christensen, H., Griffiths, K. M., & Farrer, L. (2009). Adherence in internet interventions for anxiety and depression: A systematic review. *Journal of Medical Internet Research, 11*(2), 313. Retrieved from http://www.jmir.org/2009/2/e13/

Critchfield, T. C., Tucker, J.A., & Vuchinich, R. E. (1998). Self-report methods. In K. S. Lattal & M. Perone (Eds.), *Handbook of methods in the experimental analysis of human behavior* (pp. 435–470). New York, NY: Pergamon Press.

Cummings, N. A., O'Donohue, W. T., & Ferguson, K. E. (Eds.). (2002). *Healthcare Utilization and Cost Series: Vol. 5. The impact of medical cost offset on practice and research: Making it work for you.* Reno, NV: Context Press.

Cummings, N. A., O'Donohue, W. T., & Ferguson, K. E. (Eds.). (2003). *Healthcare Utilization and Cost Series: Vol. 6. Behavioral health as primary care: Beyond efficacy to effectiveness.* Reno, NV: Context Press.

Den Boer, P. C. A. M., Wiersma, D., & Van Den Bosch, R. J. (2004). Why is self-help neglected in the treatment of emotional disorders? A meta-analysis. *Psychological Medicine, 34,* 959–971.

Edberg, M. C. (2009). *Essential readings in health behavior.* Sudbury, MA: Jones & Bartlett Publishers.

Fishbein, M., & Ajzen, I. (1975*). Belief, attitude, intention, and behavior: An introduction to theory and research.* Reading, MA: Addison-Wesley.

Flay, B. R. (1986). Efficacy and effectiveness trials (and other phases of research) in the development of health promotion programs. *Preventive Medicine, 15,* 451–474.

Fleming, M. F., Mundt, M. P., French, M. T., Manwell, L. B., Stauffacher, E. A., & Barry, K. L. (2002). Brief physician advice for problem drinkers: Long-term efficacy and benefit-cost analysis. *Alcoholism: Clinical and Experimental Research, 26,* 36–43.

Fogg, B. J. (2009). Increasing persuasion through mobility. In B. J. Fogg & D. Eckles (Eds.), *Mobile persuasion*: 20 *perspectives on the future of behavior change.* Stanford, CA: Captology Media.

Franklin, V., Wallet, A., Pagliari, C., & Greene, S. (2006). A randomized controlled trial of SweetTalk, a text-messaging service (SMS). *Diabetes Medicine, 23,* 1332–1338.

Friis, T. A., & Sellers, R. H. (2003). *Epidemiology for Public Health Practice (3rd ed.).* Sudbury, MA: Jones & Bartlett Publishers.

Glanz, K., Rimer, B. K., & Viswanath, K. J. (Eds.). (2008). *Health behavior and health education: Theory, research, and practice* (4th ed.). San Francisco, CA: Jossey-Bass.

Glasgow, R. E., Christensen, S., Smith, K. S., Stevens, V. J., & Toobert, D. J. (2009). Development and implementation of an integrated, multi-modality, user-centered interactive dietary change program. *Health Education and Research, 3,* 461–471.

Glasgow, R. E., Klesges, L. M., Dzewaltowski, D. A., Estabrooks, P. A., & Vogt, T. M. (2006). Evaluating the impact of health promotion programs using the RE-AIM framework to form summary measures for decision making involving complex issues. *Health Education Research, 21,* 688–694.

Graham, A. L., & Abrams, D. B. (2005). Reducing the cancer burden of lifestyle factors: Opportunities and challenges of the Internet. *Journal of Medical Internet Research, 7,* 26.

Green J. (2000). The role of theory in evidence-based health promotion practice. *Health Education Research, 15,* 125–129.

Greist J. H., Marks, I. M., Baer, L., Kobak K. A., Wenzel, K.W., Hirsch, M. J., ... Clary, C.M. (2002). Behavior therapy for obsessive-compulsive disorder guided by a computer or by a clinician compared with relaxation as a control. *Journal of Clinical Psychiatry, 63,* 138–145.

Grier, S., & Bryant, C. A. (2005). Social marketing in public health. *Annual Review of Public Health, 26,* 319–339.

Grimley, D. M., & Hook, E. W. (2009). A 15-minute interactive, computerized condom use intervention with biological endpoints. *Sexually Transmitted Diseases, 36,* 73–78.

Grimley, D. M., Prochaska, G. E., & Prochaska, J. O. (1997). Condom use adoption and continuation: A transtheoretical approach. *Health Education Research, 12,* 61–75.

Guttman, N. (2003). Ethics in health communication interventions. In T. L. Thompson, A. M. Dorsey, K. I. Miller, & R. Parrott (Eds.), *Handbook of health communication* (pp. 651–679). Mahwah, NJ: Lawrence Erlbaum Associates.

Harrison, J. A., Mullen, P. D., & Green, L. W. (1992). A meta-analysis of studies of the health belief model. *Health Education Quarterly, 7,* 107–116.

Hayes, S. C., & Cavoir, N. (1980). Multiple tracking and the reactivity of self-monitoring: II. Positive behaviors. *Behavioral Assessment, 2,* 283–296.

Helzer, J. E., Kraemer, H. C., Krueger, R. F., Wittchen, H.-U., Kraemer, H. C., Sirowatka, P. J., & Regier, D. A. (Eds.). (2008). *Dimensional approaches in diagnostic classification: Refining the research agenda for DSM-V.* Arlington, VA: American Psychiatric Publishing.

Helzer, J. E., Rose, G. L., Badger, G. J., Searles, J. S., Colleen, S. T., Lindberg, S. A., & Guth, S. (2008). Using interactive voice response to enhance brief alcohol intervention in primary care settings. *Journal of Studies on Alcohol and Drugs, 69,* 251–258.

Holtz, B., & Whitten, P. (2009). Managing asthma with mobile phones: A feasibility study. *Telemedicine & e-Health, 15,* 907–909.

Humphreys, K., & Tucker, J. A. (2002). Toward more responsive and effective intervention systems for alcohol-related problems. *Addiction, 97,* 126–132.

Institute of Medicine (1994). *Reducing risks for mental disorders: Frontiers for preventive intervention research.* Washington, DC: National Academies Press.

Institute of Medicine (2001). *Crossing the quality chasm: A new health care system for the 21st century.* Washington, DC: National Academies Press.

Institute of Medicine (2003). *Who will keep the public healthy? Educating public health professionals for the 21st century.* Washington, DC: National Academies Press.

Institute of Medicine (2006). *Improving the quality of health care for mental and substance-use conditions.* Washington, DC: National Academies Press.

Johnson, S. S., Driskel, M. M., Johnson, J. L., Prochaska, J. M., Zwick, W., & Prochaska, J. O. (2006). Efficacy of a transtheoretical-based expert system for antihypertensive adherence. *Disease Management, 9,* 291–301.

Joseph, J., Breslin, C., & Skinner, H. (1999). Critical perspectives on the transtheoretical model and stages of change. In J. A. Tucker, D. M. Donovan, & G. A. Marlatt (Eds.), *Changing addictive behavior: Bridging clinical and public health strategies* (pp. 160–190). New York, NY: Guilford Press..

Kay-Lambkin, F. J., Baker, A. L., Lewin, T. J., & Carr, V. J. (2009). Computer-based psychological treatment for comorbid depression and problematic alcohol and/or cannabis use: A randomized controlled trial of clinical efficacy. *Addiction, 104,* 378–388.

Kenardy, J. A., Dow, M. G. T., Johnson, D. W., Newman, M. G., Thompson, A., & Taylor, C. B. (2003). A comparison of delivery methods of cognitive behavioral therapy for panic disorder: An international multicentre trial. *Journal of Consulting and Clinical Psychology, 71,* 1068–1075.

Klingemann, H., & Sobell, L. C. (Eds.) (2007). *Promoting self-change from addictive behaviors: Practical implications for policy, prevention, and treatment.* New York, NY: Springer.

Koshy, E., Car, J., & Majeed, A. (2008). Effectiveness of mobile-phone short message service (SMS) reminders for ophthalmology outpatient appointments: Observational study. *BMC Ophthalmology, 31,* 8–9.

Kreuter, M., Farrell, D., Olevitch, L., & Brennan, L. (2000). *Tailoring health messages: Customizing communication with computer technology.* Mahwah, NJ: Lawrence Erlbaum.

Kreuter, M. W., Strecher, J. J., & Glassman, B. (1999). One size does not fit all: The case for tailoring print materials. *Annals of Behavioral Medicine, 4,* 276–283.

Krishna, S., & Boren, S.A. (2008). Diabetes self-management care via cell phone: A systematic review. *Journal of Diabetes Science and Technology, 2,* 509–517.

Krishna, S., Boren S. A., & Balas, E. A. (2009). Healthcare via cell phones: a systematic review. *Telemedicine and e-Health, 15,* 231–240.

Krueger, R. A., & Casey, M. A. (2008). *Focus groups: A practical guide for applied research* (4th ed.). Thousand Oaks, CA: Sage Publications.

Leviton, L. (1996). Integrating psychology and public health: Challenges and opportunities. *American Psychologist, 51,* 42–51.

Lieberman, J. A. (2003). History of the use of antidepressants in primary care. *Primary Care Companion Journal of Clinical Psychiatry, 5*(Suppl 7), 6–10.

Loewenstein, G. (2005a). Hot-cold empathy gaps and medical decision making. *Health Psychology, 24,* S49–S56.

Loewenstein G. (2005b). Projection bias in medical decision making. *Medical Decision Making, 25,* 96–104.

Loewenstein G., Brennan T., & Volpp, K. (2007). Asymmetric paternalism to improve health behaviors. *Journal of the American Medical Association, 298,* 2415–2417.

Madden, G. J., & Bickel, W. K. (Eds.). (2010). *Impulsivity: The behavioral and neurological science of discounting.* Washington, DC: APA Books.

Mahoney, D. F., Tarlow, B. J., & Jones, R. N. (2003). Effects of an automated telephone support system on caregiver burden and anxiety: Findings from the REACH for TLC intervention study. *Gerontologist, 43,* 556–567.

Martin, S. (2009). Improving diagnosis worldwide. *Monitor on Psychology, 40,* 62–63.

McConnaughy, E. A., Prochaska, J. O., & Velicer, W. F. (1983). Stages of change in psychotherapy: Measurement and sample profiles. *Psychotherapy: Theory, Research and Practice, 20,* 368–375.

McGuire, W. J. (1983). A contextualist theory of knowledge: Its implications for innovations and reform in psychological research. In L. Berkowitz (Ed.), *Advances in experiential social psychology* (Vol. 16, pp. 2–43). Burlington, MA: Elsevier.

McGuire, W. J. (1984). Public communication as a strategy for inducing health-promoting behavioral change. *Preventive Medicine, 13,* 299–313.

Mechanic, D. (1994). *Inescapable decisions: The imperatives of health reform.* New Brunswick, NJ: Transaction Publishers.

Miller, W. R., & Rollnick, S. (2002). *Motivational interviewing: Preparing people for change* (2nd ed.). New York, NY: Guilford Press.

Miller, W. R., & Wilbourne, P. L. (2002). Mesa Grande: A methodological analysis of clinical trials of treatments for alcohol use disorders. *Addiction, 97,* 265–277.

Muhib, F. B., Lin, L. S., Stueve, A., Miller, R. L., Ford, W. L., Johnson, W. D., & Smith, P. J. (2001). A venue-based method for sampling hard-to-reach populations. *Public Health Reports, 116* (Suppl 1), 216–222.

Mundt, J. C., Moore, H. K., & Bean, P. (2006). An interactive voice response program to reduce drinking relapse: A feasibility study. *Journal of Substance Abuse Treatment, 30,* 21–29.

Murphy, J. G., Benson, T. Vuchinich, R. E., Deskins, M., Eakin, D., Flood, A. M., ... Torrealday, O. (2004). A comparison of personalized feedback for college student drinkers delivered with and without a counseling session. *Journal of Studies on Alcohol, 65,* 200–204.

Napper, L. E., Wood, M. M., Jaffe, A., Fisher, D. G., Reynolds, G. L., & Klahn, J. A. (2008). Convergent and discriminant validity of three measures of stage of change. *Psychology of Addictive Behaviors, 22, 362–371.*

National Cancer Institute. (2001). *Making Health Communication Programs Work.* Bethesda, MD: NCI, National Institutes of Health, US Department of Health and Human Services. Retrieved from http://www.cancer.gov/pinkbook

National Cancer Institute. (2003). *Theory at a glance: A guide for health promotion practice* (2nd ed.). (NIH Publication No. 05-3896). Bethesda, MD: US Department of Health and Human Services. Retrieved from http://www.cancer.gov/PDF/481f5d53-63df-41bc-bfaf-5aa48ee1da4d/TAAG3.pdf

National Institutes of Health (2009). *NIH science of behavior change meeting summary.* Retrieved from http://nihroadmap.nih.gov/documents/SOBC_meeting_summary_2009.pdf

National Institute on Alcohol Abuse and Alcoholism. (2005). *Helping patients who drink too much: A clinician's guide.* Rockville, MD: NIAAA, National Institutes of Health, US Department of Health and Human Services. Retrieved from http://pubs.niaaa.nih. gov/publications/Practioners/CliniciansGuide2005/clinicians-guide.htm

Naylor, M. R., Keefe, F. J., Brigidi, B., Naud, S., & Helzer, J. E. (2008). Therapeutic interactive voice response for chronic pain reduction and relapse prevention. *Pain, 134,* 335–445.

Negotia, U. N. (1985). *Expert systems and fuzzy systems.* Menlo Park, CA: Benjamin/ Cummings.

Noar, S. M., Benac, C. N., & Harris, M. S. (2007). Does tailoring matter? Meta-analytic review of tailored print health behavior change interventions. *Psychological Bulletin, 133,* 673–693.

Noar, S. M., Black, H. G., & Pierce, L. B. (2009). Efficacy of computer technology-based HIV prevention interventions: A meta-analysis. *AIDS, 23*(1)*,* 107–115.

Oldenburg, B., & Glanz, K. (2008). Diffusion of innovations. In K. Glanz, B. K. Rimer, & K. J. Viswanath (Eds.), *Health behavior and health education: Theory, research, and practice* (pp. 313–333). San Francisco, CA: John Wiley & Sons.

Patrick, K., Eaab, F., Adams, M. A., Dillion, L., Zabinski, M, Rock, C. L, ... Norman, G. J. (2009). A text message-based intervention for weight loss: Randomized controlled trial. *Journal of Medical Internet Research, 11,* e1. Retrieved from http://www.jmir.org.

Pew Internet & American Life Project (2009). Wireless Internet Use, July, 2009. Retrieved from http://www. pewinternet.org/Reports/2009/12-Wireless-Internet-Use.aspx

Pini, S., Perkonnig, A., Tansella, M., & Wittchen, H. U. (1999). Prevalence and 12-month outcome of threshold and subthreshold mental disorders in primary care. *Journal of Affective Disorders, 56,* 37–48.

Plescia, M., Herrick, H., & Chavis, L. (2008). Improving health behaviors in an African-American community: The Charlotte racial and ethnic approaches to community health project. *American Journal of Public Health, 98,* 1678–1684.

Prochaska, J. O., & DiClemente, C. C. (1984). *The transtheoretical approach: Crossing traditional boundaries of therapy.* Homewood, IL: Down Jones Irwin.

Prochaska, J. O., DiClemente, C. C., & Norcross, J. C. (1992). In search of how people change: Applications to addictive behaviors, *American Psychologist, 47,* 1102–1114.

Prochaska, J. O., DiClemente, C. C., Velicer, W. R., & Rossi, J. S. (1993). Standardized, individualized, interactive, and personalized self-help programs for smoking cessation. *Health Psychology, 12,* 399–405.

Rachlin, H. (1995). Self-control: Beyond commitment. *The Behavioral and Brain Sciences, 18,* 109–159.

Reed, G. M., Lux, J. B., Bufka, L. F., Trask, C., Peterson, D. B., Stark, S., ... Hawley, J. A. (2005). Operationalizing the International Classification of Functioning, Disability and Health (ICF) in clinical settings. *Rehabilitation Psychology, 50,* 122–131.

Rodgers, A., Corbett, T., Riddell, T., Willis, M., Lin, R., & Jones, M. (2005). Do u smoke after txt? Results of a randomized trial of smoking cessation using mobile phones text messaging. *Tobacco Control, 14,* 255–261.

Rogers, E. M. (2003). *Diffusion of innovations* (3rd ed.). New York, NY: Free Press.

Rollnick, S., Miller, W. R., & Butler, C. C. (2008). *Motivational interviewing in health care: Health patients change behavior.* New York, NY: Guilford Press.

Rosenstock, I. M. (1974). Historical origins of the health belief model. *Health Education Monographs, 2,* 328–335.

Schroder, K. E. E., & Johnson, C. J. (2009). Interactive voice response technology to measure HIV-related behavior. *Current HIV/AIDS Reports, 6,* 210–216.

Seligman, M. E. P. (1995). The effectiveness of psychotherapy: The *Consumer Reports* study. *American Psychologist, 50,* 965–974.

Semple, S. J., Patterson, T. L., & Grant, I. (2000). Partner type and sexual risk behavior among HIV positive gay and bisexual men: Social cognitive correlates. *AIDS Education and Prevention, 12,* 340–356.

Sobell, L. C., Sobell, M. B., Leo, G., Agrawal, S., Johnson-Young, L., & Cunningham, J. A. (2002). Promoting self-change with alcohol abusers: A community-based mail intervention based on natural recovery studies. *Alcoholism: Clinical and Experimental Research, 26*, 936–948.

Sobell, M. B., & Sobell, L. C. (2000). Stepped care as a heuristic approach to the treatment of alcohol problems. *Journal of Consulting and Clinical Psychology, 68*, 573–579.

Strathman, A., Gleicher, F., Boninger, D. S., & Edwards, C. S. (1994). The consideration of future consequences: Weighing immediate and distant outcomes of behavior. *Journal of Personality and Social Psychology, 66*, 742–752.

Suggs, L. S., & McIntyre, C. (2007). Are we there yet? An examination of online tailored health communication. *Health Education and Behavior, 36*, 278–288.

Taylor, C. B., & Luce, K. H. (2003). Computer- and internet- based psychotherapy interventions. *Current Directions in Psychological Science, 12*, 18–22.

Tucker, J. A., & Davison, J. W. (2000). Waiting to see the doctor: The role of time constraints in the utilization of health and behavioral health services. In W. K. Bickel & R. E. Vuchinich (Eds.), *Reframing health behavior change with behavioral economics* (pp. 219–264). Mahweh, NJ: Lawrence Erlbaum.

Tucker, J. A., Foushee, H. R., & Simpson, C. A. (2009). Increasing the appeal and utilization of substance abuse services: What consumers and their social networks prefer. *International Journal of Drug Policy, 20*, 76–84.

Tucker, J. A., Murphy, J. G., & Kertesz, S. G. (2010a). Substance use disorders. In M. M. Antony & D. H. Barlow (Eds.), *Handbook of assessment, treatment planning, and outcome evaluation: Empirically supported strategies for psychological disorders* (2nd edition) (pp. 529–570). New York, NY: Guilford Press.

Tucker, J. A., Phillips, M. M., Murphy, J. G., & Raczynski, J. M. (2004). Behavioral epidemiology and health psychology. In R. G. Frank, A. Baum, & J. Wallander (Eds.), *Handbook of Clinical Health Psychology: Vol. 3. Models and perspectives in health psychology* (pp. 435–464). Washington, DC: APA Books.

Tucker, J. A., & Simpson, C. A. (in press). The recovery spectrum: From self-change to seeking treatment. *Alcohol Research and Health.*

Tucker, J. A., Simpson, C. A., & Khodneva, Y. (2010b). The role of time and delay in health decision making. In G. J. Madden & W. K. Bickel (Eds.), *Impulsivity: The behavioral and neurological science of discounting* (pp. 243–272). Washington, DC: APA Books.

US Preventive Services Task Force (2004). Screening and behavioral counseling interventions in primary care to reduce alcohol misuse: recommendation statement. *Annals of Internal Medicine, 140*, 554–556.

US Preventive Services Task Force (2009). Screening for breast cancer: U.S. Preventive Services Task Force recommendation statement. *Annals of Internal Medicine, 151*, 716–726.

US Surgeon General (1999). *Mental health: A report of the Surgeon General.* Rockville, MD: US Department of Health and Human Services, Substance Abuse and Mental Health Services Administration, Center for Mental Health Services, National Institutes of Health.

Wantland, D., Portillo C. J., Holzemer W. L., Slaughter, R., & McGhee, E. M. (2004). The effectiveness of web-based vs. non-web-based interventions: a meta-analysis of behavioral outcomes. *Journal of Medical Internet Research, 6*, e40.

Wang, P. S., Lane, M., Olfson, M., Pincus, H. A., Wells, K. B., & Kessler, R. C. (2005). Twelve-month use of mental health services in the United States: Results from the National Comorbidity Survey replication. *Archives of General Psychiatry, 62*, 629–640.

Webb, T. L., Joseph, J., Yardley, L., & Michie, S. (2010). Using the Internet to promote health behaviour change: A meta-analytic review of the impact of theoretical basis, use of behaviour change techniques, and mode of delivery on efficacy. *Journal of Medical Internet Research, 12*(1), e4. Retrieved from http://www.jmir.org/2010/1/e4

Weinreich, N. K. (1999). *Hands-on social marketing: A step-by-step guide.* Thousand Oaks, CA: Sage Publications.

WHO World Mental Health Survey Consortium (2004). Prevalence, severity, and unmet need for treatment of mental disorders in the World Health Organization Mental Health Surveys. *Journal of the American Medical Association, 291*, 2581–2590.

Witte, K., & Allen, M. (2000). A meta-analysis of fear appeals: Implications for effective public health campaigns. *Health Education & Behavior, 27*, 591–615.

Wong, F., Huhman, M., Heitzler, C., Asbury, L., Bretthauer-Mueller, R., McCarthy, S., & Londe, P. (2004). VERB™ – a social marketing campaign to increase physical activity among youth. *Prevention of Chronic Disease* [serial online]*, 2004 July* [date cited]. Retrieved from http://www.cdc.gov/pcd/issues/2004/jul/04_0043.htm

Zimbardo, P., & Boyd, J. (2008). *The time paradox: The new psychology of time that will change your life*. New York, NY: Free Press.

8

Appendices: Tools and Resources

This chapter contains resources that providers can copy and use (items are presented in the order in which they are discussed in the chapters):

Appendix 1: Consideration of Future Consequences (CFC) Scale

For each of the statements below, please indicate whether or not the statement is characteristics of you. If the statement is extremely uncharacteristic of you (not at all like you), please write a "1" to the left of the question: if the statement is extremely characteristic of you (very much like you) please write a "5" next to the question. And, of course, use the numbers in the middle if you fall between the extremes. Please keep the following scale in mind as you rate each of the statements below.

1 = extremely uncharacteristic	2 = somewhat uncharacteristic	3 = uncertain/ neutral	4 = somewhat characteristic	5 = extremely characteristic

_____ 1. I consider how things might be in the future, and try to influence those things in my day-to-day behavior.

_____ 2. Often I engage in a particular behavior in order to achieve outcomes that may not result for many years.

_____ 3. I only act to satisfy immediate concerns, figuring the future will take care of itself.

_____ 4. My behavior is only influenced by immediate (i.e., a matter of days or weeks) outcomes of my actions.

_____ 5. My convenience is a big factor in the decisions I make or the actions I take.

_____ 6. I am willing to sacrifice my immediate happiness or well-being in order to achieve future outcomes.

_____ 7. I think it is important to take warnings about negative outcomes seriously even if the negative outcome will not occur for many years.

_____ 8. I think it is more important to perform a behavior with important distant consequences than a behavior with less important immediate consequences.

_____ 9. I generally ignore warnings about possible future problems because I think the problems will be resolved before they reach crisis level.

_____ 10. I think that sacrificing now is usually unnecessary since future outcomes can be dealt with at a later time.

_____ 11. I only act to satisfy immediate concerns, figuring that I will take care of future problems that may occur at a later date.

_____ 12. Since my day-to-day work has specific outcomes, it is more important to me than behavior that has distant outcomes.

CFC Scoring: Items 1, 2, 6, 7, and 8 are scored as answered. Items 3, 4, 5, 9, 10, 11, and 12 are reverse scored. Higher scores demonstrate greater future time orientation. Copyright © 1994 by the American Psychological Association. Adapted with permission from "The Consideration of Future Consequences: Weighing Immediate and Distant Outcomes of Behavior," by A. Strathman, F. Gleicher, D. S. Boninger, & C. S. Edwards, 1994, _Journal of Personality and Social Psychology, 66,_ 742–752.

Appendix 2: Self-Monitoring and Guided Self-Change Materials

Substance Use Disorders

http://www2.potsdam.edu/alcohol-info/DrinkTooMuch.html
"Drink Too Much?" emphasizes practical ways of moderating alcohol consumption.

http://www.med.umich.edu/drinkwise
Drink Wise is a brief intervention for persons seeking to eliminate negative consequences of mild to moderate problem drinking.

http://www.moderation.org
Moderation Management is oriented to moderation drinking and self-management.

https://ncadistore.samhsa.gov/catalog/referrals.aspx?topic=83&h=resources
The National Clearinghouse for Alcohol and Drug Information (NCADI) links to information and resources.

http://www.rational.org/recovery
Rational Recovery is a secular organization emphasizing personal strength rather than spirituality.

http://www.secularhumanism.org/sos
Secular Organizations for Sobriety (SOS), sometimes called Save Our Selves, has a secular orientation and abstinence focus.

http://www.smartrecovery.org
Self-Management and Recovery Training (SMART Recovery) defines alcoholism as a bad habit and provides practical strategies for breaking the habit.

http://www.womenforsobriety.org
Women for Sobriety is a secular organization emphasizing self-esteem; caffeine, sugar, and tobacco are not allowed at meetings.

Sexual Risk Behaviors

http://www.thebody.com/
A service of the Body Health Resources Corporation offering a complete HIV/AIDS resource.

Time Horizons

http://www.thetimeparadox.com/
Zimbardo Time Perspective Inventory and the Transcendental-Future Time Perspective Inventory.

Depression

http://www.helpguide.org/mental/depression_tips.htm
Tips and tools for self-management of depressive symptoms and directory of online self-help resources.

http://www.dbsalliance.org/site/PageServer?pagename=home
Self-assessment information from the Depression and Bipolar Support Alliance and links to local support groups.

Anxiety

http://www.helpguide.org/mental/anxiety_self_help.htm
Tips, tools, and a directory of online self-help resources.

http://www.cci.health.wa.gov.au/resources/infopax.cfm?Info_ID=46
Eleven-module self-help course for anxiety from the Centre for Clinical Interventions, Department of Health, Western Australia.

Nutrition and Physical Activity

http://www.smallstep.gov/
Small-step initiative of the US Department of Health and Human Services.

http://www.fruitsandveggiesmatter.gov/
US Centers for Disease Control and Prevention website for the 5-A-Day program to increase fruit and vegetable consumption.

Appendix 3: Websites with Behavioral Health Intervention Materials

Substance Use Disorders

http://pubs.niaaa.nih.gov/publications/Practitioner/CliniciansGuide2005/clinicians_guide.htm
Helping Patients Who Drink Too Much: A Clinician's Guide (2005 edition) is published by the US National Institute on Alcohol Abuse and Alcoholism. The manual targets case-finding, brief intervention, and referral for primary care providers.

http://www.drugabuse.gov/nidamed/
NIDAMED resources of the US National Institute on Drug Abuse (NIDA) include videos and downloadable treatment and prevention guides, practice materials for providers, patient information guides, and youth-targeted publications.

http://www.drugabuse.gov/TB/Clinical/ClinicalToolbox.html and http://www.nidatoolbox.org/
The NIDA Clinical Toolbox offers science-based materials for providers of drug abuse treatments.

HIV/AIDS

www.effectiveinterventions.org
This US Centers for Disease Control and Prevention (CDC) site for Diffusion of Effective Behavioral Interventions (DEBI) describes evidence-based interventions to prevent transmission of HIV, other sexually transmitted infections, and viral hepatitis.

http://www.drugabuse.gov/CBOM/Index.html
This NIDA site provides a description, brochure, and a complete manual for HIV prevention using the community-based outreach model.

Mental Health

http://www.nrepp.samhsa.gov/
The US National Registry of Evidence-Based Programs and Practices (NREPP) is operated by the Substance Abuse and Mental Health Services Administration. The database covers mental health, substance abuse, HIV, and co-occurring disorders. It is searchable by condition, level of evidence, age group, etc.

Nutrition and Physical Activity

http://www.cdc.gov/wisewoman/
The CDC WISEWOMAN site provides risk factor screening, lifestyle intervention, and referrals to specialty care for low income, underinsured women of color.

http://www.cdc.gov/leanworks/
LEAN Works is a CDC program to assist employers in implementing worksite-based health promotion programs. Resources include guidelines for selecting, planning, implementing, and evaluating a program that will meet the specific company's needs.

Appendix 4: IVR Self-Monitoring to Support Natural Resolution: Sample Questions from Daily Lead and Drinking-Related Surveys

DAILY SURVEY			
Item	Introduction/Information	Question	Responses
AnswerIntro	Thank you for calling the UAB Interactive Voice Response system.	Please enter your 4-digit PIN number now.	XXXX
StudyDays	Since you have started, this is study day number [DAY]		
DaysCalled	The total number of days that you have called in is [DAYS]		
ConsecutiveDays	You have called in for the following number of consecutive days [DAYS]		
We start today with the daily questions about your drinking practices yesterday.			
BeerOunces	The first questions ask about the amount of beer, wine, and liquor that you drank yesterday.	How many ounces of beer did you drink yesterday?	0–500
WineOunces		How many ounces of wine did you drink yesterday?	0–200
LiquorOunces		How many ounces of hard liquor did you drink yesterday?	0–98
UrgeDrink	Next, whether or not you drank yesterday, rate your urge to drink yesterday.	Use any number from 0 to 9. Zero means you had no urge to drink and 9 means you had the strongest urge ever to drink.	0–9
AlcoholAvailable	Whether or not you drank yesterday, how much time did you spend in situations where others were drinking or where alcohol was available?	Enter the total minutes yesterday when alcohol was present.	0–1000
SpendAlcohol	Whether or not you drank yesterday, how much money did you spend yesterday on alcoholic beverages?	Enter the amount of money you spent in dollars. Round up or down to the nearest whole dollar. Enter zero if you spent no money.	0–2000

Appendix 5: Sample Graphs of Daily Drinking from the Preresolution Year Through Month 6 Postresolution (1 Participant)

Description for participants: The graph below shows your daily alcohol intake during the year before you stopped problem drinking to the present. It is based on your reports during the initial interview and then using the interactive voice response (IVR) system. Day 365 is the day you stopped problem drinking. Daily alcohol intake is shown in standard drinks (12 oz. beer, 5 oz. wine, or 1.5 oz. liquor).

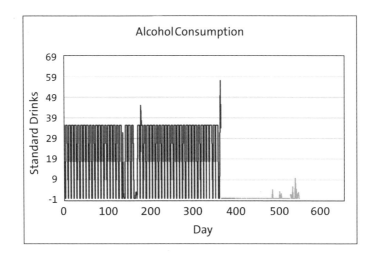

Description for participants: We have enlarged your IVR reports of daily drinking since you started recording. This will let you see the extent to which you are staying within your personal drinking limits and within the limits recommended by the National Institute on Alcohol Abuse and Alcoholism (NIAAA) (no more than 14 drinks per week for men and 7 drinks per week for women, and each week should include some abstinent days). NIAAA further recommends that men never consume more than 4 drinks in a single day and that women never consume more than 3 drinks in a single day. This means you want to stay below the **unsafe drinking zone**.

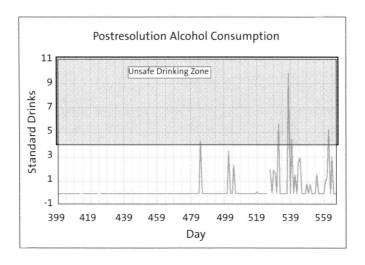

Appendix 6: Best Practices Guidelines for IVR Behavioral Health Applications

Abu-Hasaballah et al. (2007, pp. 600–601) offer the following "best practices" guidelines based on their review of interactive voice response (IVR) medical studies:

- *Script design* – Eliminate any features that promote inaccurate or incomplete reports.
- *IVR script validation* – Necessary to insure that assessment or intervention procedures established as evidence-based in other formats work satisfactorily using the IVR format.
- *IVR script piloting* – Do this with a few callers before full implementation, to identify and remediate protocol problems (e.g., poor questions or response options, improper skip and branch functions).
- *Participant training* – Prior to use of the IVR system, cover general system (e.g., toll-free number, personal identification number, keypad options) and protocol-specific (e.g., questions, response options) features.
- *Monitoring of participant compliance* – Staff should monitor calls frequently (e.g., daily) and judiciously use automatic reminder or personal calls to promote IVR use. Although prompts early in the IVR interval may help establish regular calls, persistent reminders after considerable noncompliance are not helpful (Mundt et al., 2006).

To the best practices described by Abu-Hasaballah et al. (2007), we add a few of our own based on our IVR applications:

- *Verbal report quality* – IVR reports are fundamentally verbal reports and thus are governed by the considerations and procedures identified in the assessment literature to enhance reliability and accuracy (reviewed by Critchfield, Tucker, & Vuchinich, 1998).
- *Script order and duration* – Ask more important questions early in the IVR script, and keep the entire session < 5–10 minutes maximum for an experienced caller. Otherwise, callers may end the call before they finish the assessment.
- *Question and response formatting* – When questions are repeated day after day, include key words early in the questions that allow callers to respond immediately thereafter. Vary the response options so that callers cannot enter the same number repeatedly without listening, and include programs that ask callers to reenter or affirm out-of-range or unusual responses.
- *Caller feedback and incentives* – Long-term IVR use can be promoted by including individualized verbal feedback about calling patterns as part of the IVR calls. For very long-term IVR applications (months to years), awarding points that accrue for small monetary payments or entry into a lottery for prizes or money can be used to reinforce regular calling patterns.

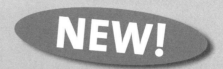

H. Russel Searight

Practicing Psychology in Primary Care

2010, iv + 160 pages, ISBN: 978-0-88937-362-4
US $29.80 / € 20.95 / £ 16.90

H. Russell Searight

Practicing Psychology in Primary Care

HOGREFE

Equips psychologists, mental health professionals, and trainees to work effectively in a primary care setting – the principal site today for psychiatric care, behavioral health risk reduction, and psychological treatment of physical or functional complaints.

The primary care setting has a "culture" that is very distinct from more traditional mental health settings, and so the first part of this book teaches both professional clinicians and students about the norms, communication styles, social rituals, and roles they need to be familiar with to be effective psychologists in primary care.

Psychological therapies in primary care must be symptom-focused and brief. A broad-based epidemiological perspective is also necessary to address mood and anxiety disorders, medical nonadherence, and health risk behaviors such as alcohol abuse and smoking among a large number of patients. Core chapters in the book therefore describe counseling techniques developed specifically for primary care such as the Four A's and BATHE, the Transtheoretical Model (TM), adaptations of Motivational Interviewing (MI) and Problem-Solving Therapy (PSA), as well as cross-cultural considerations and consultations as a mental health intervention.

Equipped with these strategies and a deeper appreciation of primary care culture, readers will be well placed to adapt their clinical skills to this challenging and rewarding health care setting.

About the Author:

H. Russell Searight is Associate Professor of Psychology at Lake Superior State University in Sault Sainte Marie, Michigan. For 18 years, he was Director of Behavioral Science at the Forest Park Hospital Family Medicine Residency and on the faculty of Saint Louis University School of Medicine. He has published three previous books and over 140 articles and book chapters.

Hogrefe Publishing
30 Amberwood Parkway · Ashland, OH 44805 · USA
Tel: (800) 228-3749 · Fax: (419) 281-6883
E-Mail: customerservice@hogrefe.com

Hogrefe Publishing
Rohnsweg 25 · 37085 Göttingen · Germany
Tel: +49 551 999 500 · Fax: +49 551 999 50 425
E-Mail: customerservice@hogrefe.de

Hogrefe Publishing c/o Marston Book Services Ltd
PO Box 269 · Abingdon, OX14 4YN · UK
Tel: +44 1235 465577 · Fax +44 1235 465556
direct.orders@marston.co.uk

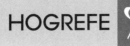

HOGREFE

Order online at **www.hogrefe.com**
or call toll-free **(800) 228-3749** (US only)

Available soon!
Reserve your copy now!

Alan L. Peterson, Mark W. Vander Weg & Carlos Roberto Jaén

Nicotine and Tobacco Dependence

In the series: Advances in Psychotherapy – Evidence-Based Practice: Volume 21

2011, ca. 104 pages, softcover
US $29.80 / € 24.95 / £ 19.90 (Series Standing Order: US $24.80 / € 19.95 / £ 15.90)
ISBN: 978-0-88937-324-2

How to stop patients and clients smoking - guidance on treatments that work, from leading US authorities.

This volume in the series *Advances in Psychotherapy: Evidence-Based Practice* provides health care providers with practical and evidence-based guidance on the diagnosis and treatment of nicotine and tobacco dependence. Tobacco use is the leading preventable cause of death in the world, and it is the only legally available consumer product that kills people when used entirely as intended. Research over the past several decades has led to the development of a number of evidence-based treatments for nicotine and tobacco dependence that can be delivered by health care professionals in a variety of primary and specialty care settings. This book aims to increase medical, mental health, and dental practitioners' access to empirically supported interventions for nicotine and tobacco dependence, with the hope that these methods will be incorporated into routine clinical practice.

The book is both a compact "how-to" reference for clinicians and an ideal educational resource for students and for practice-oriented continuing education. The volume includes tables, boxed clinical pearls, and clinical vignettes, and the appendix includes clinical tools, patient handouts, and links to the top recommended websites for the download of additional patient materials.

Alan L. Peterson · Mark W. Vander Weg · Carlos R. Jaén

Nicotine and Tobacco Dependence

Advances in Psychotherapy
Evidence-Based Practice

HOGREFE

For further details visit www.hogrefe.com

Hogrefe Publishing
30 Amberwood Parkway · Ashland, OH 44805 · USA
Tel: (800) 228-3749 · Fax: (419) 281-6883
E-Mail: customerservice@hogrefe.com

Hogrefe Publishing
Rohnsweg 25 · 37085 Göttingen · Germany
Tel: +49 551 999 500 · Fax: +49 551 999 50 425
E-Mail: customerservice@hogrefe.de

Hogrefe Publishing c/o Marston Book Services Ltd
PO Box 269 · Abingdon, OX14 4YN · UK
Tel: +44 1235 465577 · Fax +44 1235 465556
direct.orders@marston.co.uk

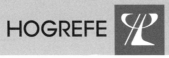

HOGREFE

Order online at **www.hogrefe.com**
or call toll-free **(800) 228-3749** (US only)

Visit **www.hogrefe.com** for more details

Advances in Psychotherapy – Evidence-Based Practice

Developed and edited with the support of the Society of Clinical Psychology (APA Division 12)

Series Editor: *Danny Wedding*
Associate Editors: *Larry E. Beutler, Kenneth E. Freedland, Linda Carter Sobell, David A. Wolfe*

Bibliographic features of each volume: ca. 80-120 pages, softcover, US $29.80 / £ 19.90 / € 24.95
Standing order price (minimum 4 successive vols.) US $24.80 / £15.90 / € 19.95
*Special rates for members of the Society of Clinical Psychology (APA D12) :
 Single volume: US $24.80 / Standing order: US $19.80 per volume
(+postage & handling)

Save 20% with a Series Standing Order

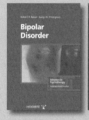
Bipolar Disorder

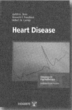
Heart Disease

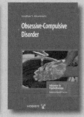
Obsessive-Compulsive Disorder

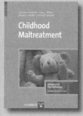
Childhood Maltreatment

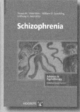
Schizophrenia

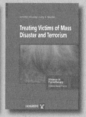
Treating Victims of Mass Disaster and Terrorism

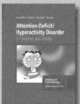
Attention-Deficit/ Hyperactivity Disorder in Children and Adults

Problem and Pathological Gambling

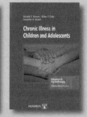
Chronic Illness in Children and Adolescents

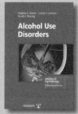
Alcohol Use Disorders

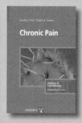
Chronic Pain

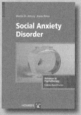
Social Anxiety Disorder

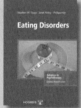
Eating Disorders

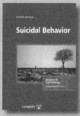
Suicidal Behavior

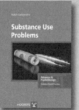
Substance Use Problems

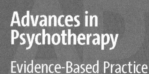
Advances in Psychotherapy
Evidence-Based Practice

NEW!

NEW!

NEW!

Coming soon!

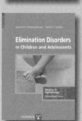
Elimination Disorders in Children and Adolescents

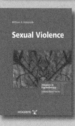
Sexual Violence

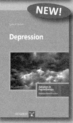
Depression

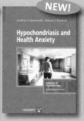
Hypochondriasis and Health Anxiety

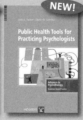
Public Health Tools for Practicing Psychologists

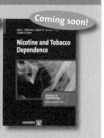
Nicotine and Tobacco Dependence

Hogrefe Publishing
30 Amberwood Parkway · Ashland, OH 44805 · USA
Tel: (800) 228-3749 · Fax: (419) 281-6883
E-Mail: customerservice@hogrefe.com

Hogrefe Publishing
Rohnsweg 25 · 37085 Göttingen · Germany
Tel: +49 551 999 500 · Fax: +49 551 999 50 425
E-Mail: customerservice@hogrefe.de

Hogrefe Publishing c/o Marston Book Services Ltd
PO Box 269 · Abingdon, OX14 4YN · UK
Tel: +44 1235 465577 · Fax +44 1235 465556
direct.orders@marston.co.uk

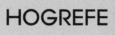

Order online at **www.hogrefe.com**
or call toll-free **(800) 228-3749** (US only)